MOMENT TO MOMENT

Perspectives on
Fetal Alcohol Spectrum
Disorders in Adolescence

Edited by
Ira J. Chasnoff, MD

nti upstream

Chicago, IL   Portland, OR

Moment to Moment: Perspectives on
Fetal Alcohol Spectrum Disorders in Adolescence

Copyright © 2014
Edited by Ira J. Chasnoff, MD

All rights reserved. Except as permitted under the U.S. Copyright Act of 1976, no part of this publication may be reproduced, distributed, or transmitted in any form, or by any means, or stored in a database or retrieval system, without the prior written permission of the publisher.

NTI Upstream
2066 NW Irving Street, Suite 1
Portland, OR 97209

Please visit www.ntiupstream.com for information about all books and other related products. For more information about discounts for bulk purchases or to schedule a live event, please email: info@ntiupstream.com.

Chapter 7: FASDs and the Justice System is excerpted in part, with permission by the publisher, Bentham e-Books, from "Chapter 7, FASD and the Law," by K.A. Kelly, from *Prenatal Alcohol Use and Fetal Alcohol Spectrum Disorders: Diagnosis, Assessment and New Directions in Research and Multimodal Treatment.*

Cover and Interior Design by Melanie Jansen-Daniels

Printed in the United States of America

Library of Congress Control Number: 2014941496
ISBN: 978-0-9707762-3-5

MOMENT
TO MOMENT

Perspectives on
Fetal Alcohol Spectrum
Disorders in Adolescence

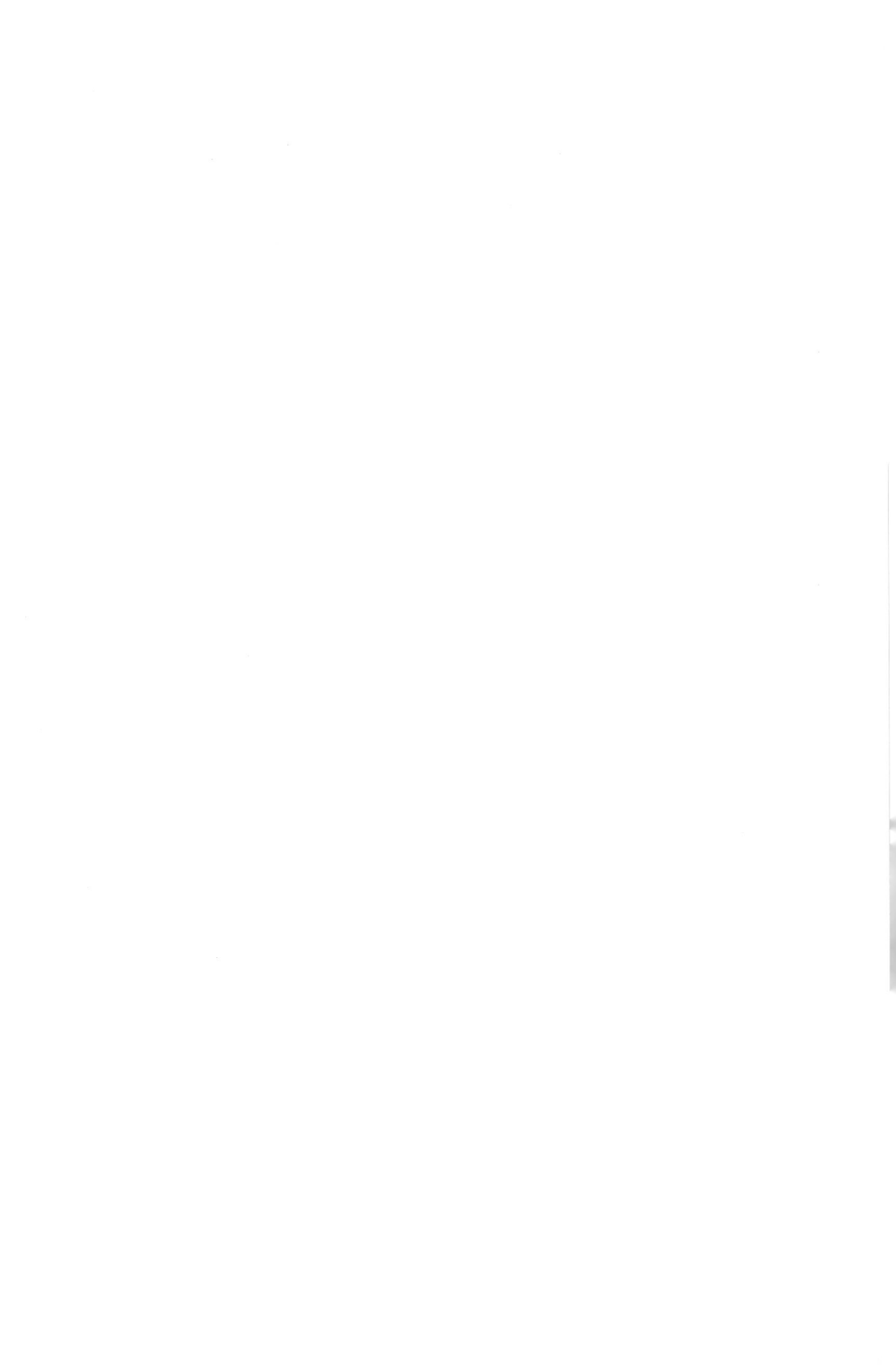

Contents

Introduction   **11**

CHAPTER 1: Medical   **15**
Fetal Alcohol Spectrum Disorders: Behavior Belongs in the Brain
Ira J. Chasnoff, M.D.

CHAPTER 2: Psychology   **39**
Fetal Alcohol Spectrum Disorders in the Teenage Years
Julie Kable, Ph.D.

CHAPTER 3: Education   **67**
FASDs, Adolescence and School
Ron Powell, Ph.D.

CHAPTER 4: Therapy   **95**
The Perfect Storm: Complexity of Sexual Behaviors
in Adolescents with FASDs
Jenae Holtz, L.M.F.T.

CHAPTER 5: Parenting   **119**
S.O.S: A Parent's Cry for Help or a Survival Strategy?
Carole Hurley, J.D.

CHAPTER 6: Child Welfare   **135**
Fetal Alcohol Spectrum Disorders, Adolescents,
and the Child Welfare System
Sidney Gardner

CHAPTER 7: Legal   **153**
FASDs and the Justice System
Howard Davidson, J.D., and Katherine Kelly

CHAPTER 8: Communications   **181**
The Dangers of Cyberspace
Ira J. Chasnoff, M.D., and Jonathan Leuchs, M.P.I.A.

Author Biographies   **193**

Discussion Questions   **199**

Introduction

Moment to Moment: Perspectives on FASDs in Adolescence is designed for families and professionals who care for children with Fetal Alcohol Spectrum Disorders. The information in this book complements the documentary of the same name and offers a more in-depth discussion of the basic facts about prenatal alcohol exposure, providing further insight into the reasons behind the children's behaviors. Experts from a variety of fields share their perspectives to the challenges we face as we care for adolescents who have been affected by their biological mothers' use of alcohol during pregnancy. Each chapter is designed to shine a new light from a variety of angles on FASDs, including the important perspective of a parent who has guided her daughter into young adulthood.

The companion film, *Moment to Moment: Growing Up with FASDs,* is the story of four adolescents and their adoptive families. The four young people suffer a wide range of disabilities – physical, emotional, and developmental – due to their prenatal exposure to alcohol. The interventions and treatment they require cover an even broader range. The families' determination, hope, dreams for their children come to the fore as the camera explores the children's life on a daily basis.

We seek to educate all who can prevent FASDs and those dedicated professionals who treat children with FASDs. But ultimately, we hope that this set of materials will help us all learn to look beyond the behaviors we see and to understand the source and purpose of those behaviors as children with FASDs struggle to deal with a world they have difficulty comprehending.

Ira J. Chasnoff, MD   *Editor*

CHAPTER 1 *Medical*

**FETAL ALCOHOL SPECTRUM DISORDERS:
BEHAVIOR BELONGS IN THE BRAIN**

Ira J. Chasnoff, M.D.

Dr. Ira J. Chasnoff, president of NTI Upstream and Professor of Clinical Pediatrics at the University of Illinois College of Medicine, provides an overview of Fetal Alcohol Spectrum Disorders and an in-depth look at how the fetal brain is affected by exposure to alcohol. He uses this information to offer an explanation of how the child's compromised nervous system is at the heart of the child's behavioral difficulties.

Over the last several decades, progress has been slow in determining how many children in this country are affected by prenatal exposure to alcohol. A combination of legal, social, and attitudinal barriers has restrained communication on every level, starting with the health care provider and patient. Physicians rarely ask a pregnant woman about her alcohol intake, and fetal alcohol syndrome (FAS) remains the most common cause of preventable intellectual disabilities in the United States as well as one of the leading causes of behavioral problems in children.

The prevalence of FAS is estimated to range from 0.2 to 2 cases per 1,000 live births, depending on ethnic, cultural, and regional factors.[1] Given the approximately 4 million births per year in the United States, there are up to 6,000 children born in this country each year with FAS. But the problem is even worse than these statistics suggest.

A recent study[2] of 100,653 pregnant women in six states documented that 31% of the women had a positive screen for substance use: 23.4% were using alcohol and 8.9% were using illicit drugs, including marijuana, narcotics, cocaine, and methamphetamine. These data are similar to results from the *2008–2009 National Survey on Drug Use and Health*.[3]

This survey, based on a national sample of women, revealed that in the first trimester 8.5% of pregnant women use illicit drugs, 20.4% drink alcohol, and 22.4% smoke cigarettes. Thus, about 1 million children across the United States may be exposed prenatally to alcohol each year. These children can suffer from a broad range of difficulties that, while often quite subtle, can compromise the children's long-term health, behavior, development, and academic achievement.[4-8]

CRITERIA FOR DIAGNOSIS

Fetal alcohol syndrome is the original name given to a cluster of physical and mental defects present from birth that are the direct result of a woman's drinking alcoholic beverages while pregnant. Infants with FAS have signs in three categories: (1) growth deficiencies, (2) central nervous system impairment, and (3) facial dysmorphology.[9]

The mother's confirmed use of alcohol is not necessary to make a diagnosis of FAS if the child meets criteria in all three categories. However, to ensure accuracy and completeness in the child's medical records, physicians should note when the diagnosis is based solely on these physical and developmental parameters and without confirmation of the mother's drinking.

As we begin this discussion, it is important to realize that the impact of prenatal alcohol exposure is not determined only by the cumulative "dose" of alcohol to which the child was exposed. Many reports demonstrate that the mother's binge drinking, with high peak blood alcohol levels, is actually more dangerous than chronic drinking. Recent studies regarding adolescents have noted that even "light drinking" during pregnancy has a significant detrimental impact on the adolescent's neurodevelopmental status.[10]

GROWTH DEFICIENCIES

In the United States, the average birth weight of babies born at term (38 to 42 weeks gestation) is 7 pounds 8 ounces, with a normal range down to 5 pounds 8 ounces. Babies born to mothers who use alcohol have an average birth weight of around 6 pounds and are more likely than babies born to mothers who abstained to weigh less than 5 pounds 8 ounces.[11] As children with fetal alcohol syndrome grow older, they tend to continue to be small for their age—that is, short and underweight. To meet the FAS diagnostic guidelines set for growth criteria, a child must have either reduced weight *or* height (at or below 10th percentile on standard growth charts) at birth *or* at any point in time after birth.[11]

CHANGES IN FACIAL FEATURES

Facial features associated with prenatal alcohol exposure are consistent with mid-face hypoplasia, an overall undergrowth with resultant flattening of the middle portion of the face. Thus, children with FAS exhibit:

- Epicanthal folds (extra skin folds coming down around the inner angle of the eye)
- Short palpebral fissures (small eye openings)
- A flattened elongated philtrum (no groove or crease running from the bottom of the nose to the top of the lip)
- Thin upper lip
- Small mouth with high arched palate (roof of the mouth)
- Small teeth with poor enamel coating
- Low set ears.[9,11]

FACIES IN FETAL ALCOHOL SYNDROME

FIG 1.1

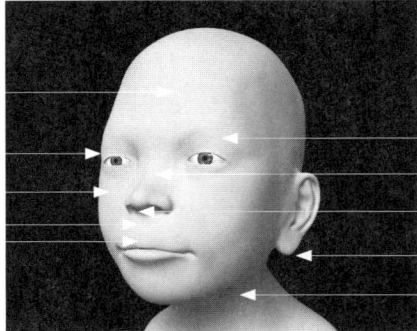

Microcephaly
Short palpebral fissures
Flattened midface
Flat philtrum
Thin upper lip

Epicanthal folds
Flat nasal bridge
Short, upturned nose
Low set ears
Receding jaw

These changes can vary in severity, but usually persist over the life of the child. Most people will not recognize any differences when they see the child, but physicians and other practitioners with experience in working with children prenatally exposed to alcohol will be able to detect the changes.

A problem arises when clinicians rely too heavily on changes in facial structure to recognize the child affected by prenatal alcohol exposure. In animal studies, pregnant rats given alcohol on days 7 or 8 after conception had newborns with facial features typical of FAS. However, giving the pregnant rats alcohol on days 1 through 6, or on day 9 or any time beyond did not affect the facial features in any way. Thus, there appears to be a very narrow window of alcohol exposure that can affect children's facial features.

Children with prenatal alcohol exposure also may have a variety of malformations of major organs, especially the heart, kidneys, eyes, and ears.[9,11] Children with prenatal alcohol exposure frequently have vision problems; many have an eye that turns inward (i.e., esotropia, or a "lazy eye"). In addition, the children can have a predisposition to ear infections and a high rate of partial or complete hearing loss (i.e., eighth nerve deafness), so a thorough hearing exam is recommended in the first year of life and should be repeated based on the child's speech and language development.

CENTRAL NERVOUS SYSTEM IMPAIRMENT

Problems in the central nervous system can become manifest through structural, neurological, or functional changes.[4,11] Structurally, a small head circumference (at or below 10th percentile) at birth or at any time thereafter indicates poor brain growth. For example, the average head size of term infants at birth is 35 centimeters, while the head size of a baby with FAS often is less than 33 centimeters. Neurological damage can be manifest as seizures, problems in coordination, difficulty with motor control, or a number of "soft" neurological deficits. Functionally, the average IQ in children with FAS is in the 70s, as compared to the general population in which the average IQ is 100. Alcohol-exposed children, with or without the characteristic facial features or growth retardation, have consistently lower IQ scores than non-exposed children. Importantly, even alcohol-exposed children with a "normal IQ" demonstrate difficulty with behavioral regulation, impulsivity, social deficits, and poor judgment, causing problems in day-to-day management in the classroom and home.

Children affected by prenatal alcohol exposure exhibit a wide range of functional difficulties much more commonly than global intellectual impairment; these difficulties include learning disabilities, poor school performance, diminished executive functioning (e.g., organization of tasks, understanding cause and effect, following several steps of directions), clumsiness, poor balance, and problems with writing or drawing. Behaviorally, many of the children have a short attention span, and often are described as impulsive and hyperactive. [5,7,8,13,14]

From a brain structure perspective, prenatal alcohol exposure not only can cause the child to have a small brain overall but also can stunt the growth of individual parts of the brain.[4,11,15] This damaged growth may be present regardless of the child's facial features. Problems with the formation and development of different parts of the brain can result in a wide range of behavioral and learning deficits. Many children and adolescents with prenatal alcohol exposure have trouble moving information between different brain regions; they cannot effectively use information to self-direct their behavior or to think in the abstract. They may have trouble learning new information and recording it in the brain—and then have even more difficulty retrieving the information they've already learned. A child may learn his multiplication tables one day, but forget them the next.

Other parts of the brain also can be affected, impairing the child's ability to coordinate planned motor movements and resulting in impulsive movement and clumsiness.[4,15]

Reduction in the size of the cerebellum in the back part of the brain, for example, produces difficulties with balance and arousal and may be a source of sleep problems. Again, it is important to remember that such problems occur not only in children with the abnormal facial features associated with full expression of FAS, but also in alcohol-exposed children who "look normal."

BRAIN STRUCTURE AND FUNCTION: DEFICITS IN INFORMATION PROCESSING

The behavioral, emotional, and learning difficulties of children with prenatal alcohol exposure can be best understood as a deficit in processing information.[7,12,13,16] More specifically, children have difficulty recording information (bringing it into the brain); interpreting information; storing information in memory for later use; and using information to guide actions, behavior, emotions, language, and movement. The normal MRI shown in Figure 1.2 demonstrates some key brain structures and areas affected by drug and alcohol exposure. The cerebral cortex is the outer shell of the brain; the prefrontal cortex is a component of the overall cortex, the area that contains dopamine and serves as the regulatory center of the brain; the corpus callosum is a part of the limbic system, located in the exact midline of the brain.

NORMAL MRI OF BRAIN

FIG 1.2

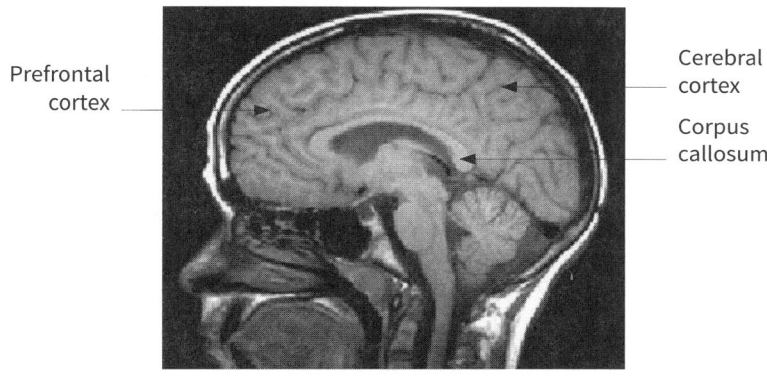

Prefrontal cortex

Cerebral cortex

Corpus callosum

Damage from drinking in the first trimester—that is, the first three months of pregnancy—mainly occurs in the midline structures of the brain, where the limbic system is located. The limbic system guides information processing: the way we bring information into the brain and use it to manage our behaviors, emotions, and thoughts. As seen in Figure 1.3, data retrieved from our senses enter the brain through different pathways. Visual information enters through the back portion of the brain, a region known as the occipital lobe. Touch, taste, and smell enter through the parietal lobe, located in the upper, posterior half of the brain. Auditory information enters through the ear, and the eighth cranial nerve carries the information from the ear to the inner midline section of the brain.

PATHWAYS FOR BRINGING INFORMATION INTO THE BRAIN

FIG 1.3

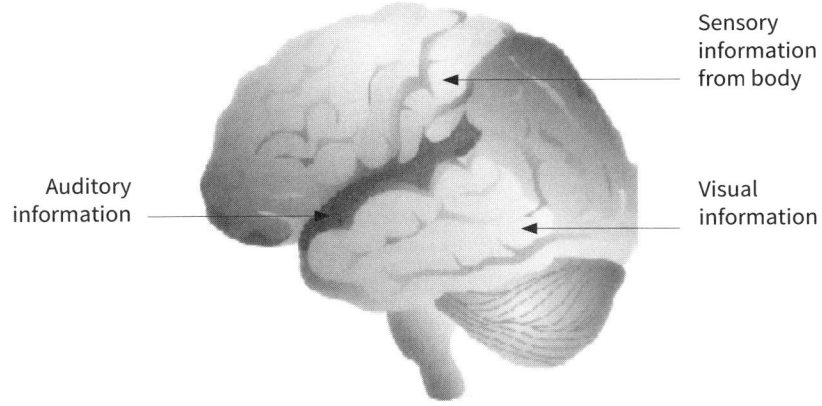

A primary job of the brain is to bring these disparate bits of sensory input together and conduct the information to the prefrontal cortex in the front of the brain. There, dopamine, a key neurotransmitter, is fired off at intervals to guide the individual in using and responding appropriately to the information via motor activity, behavior, emotion, speech and language. In other words, by regulating the amount and frequency of dopamine release, the individual is able to use information *from* the environment to manage a response *to* the environment.

Alcohol's damage to the limbic system is what produces many of the functional difficulties we see in children exposed prenatally to alcohol. For example, the hippocampus, situated in the posterior aspect of the limbic system, plays a role in consolidating new memories and applying information in novel situations. If the hippocampus is damaged, the child has difficulty transferring neurologically generated maps of information and experience to long-term memory storehouses in the temporal lobes. The child may know, cognitively, not to run out into a particular street in front of his house, but cannot retrieve that knowledge when approaching a different street. As a result, he runs out into the street, appearing to be "impulsive" or "hyperactive."

Other alcohol-induced structural changes in the brain can occur in the corpus callosum, the portion of the brain that permits the two major halves to share information. When compared to the normal MRI seen previously (Figure 1.2), the corpus callosum in the MRI of the child with FAS (Figure 1.4) is narrower at its posterior segment. This structural thinning effect disrupts communication within the brain so that certain types of information can never reach consciousness. For example, an alcohol-exposed child may be able to recite the rules for good behavior in the school lunchroom, but be unable to regulate his behavior in accordance with those rules. As a result, he is described as disobedient or labeled with a diagnosis of oppositional defiant disorder (ODD): "He knows what he's supposed to do," exclaims his teacher. "He just won't do it!" Although a child with FAS may meet diagnostic criteria for oppositional defiant disorder, diagnostic and therapeutic approaches must consider the nature of the structural brain defects that are producing the behavior before such a determination is made. We are asking clinicians and parents to look beyond the behavior they see to identify the root cause of that behavior.

THINNING OF THE CORPUS CALLOSUM IN A CHILD WITH FAS

FIG 1.4

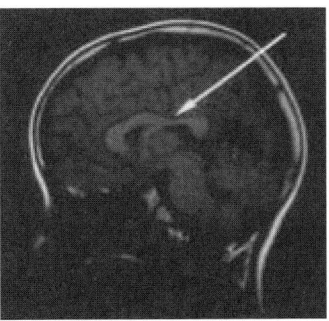

As another example, the thalamus (also part of the limbic system) receives input from all over the body and sends it to the cerebral cortex, the area of the brain responsible for cognition and learning. The thalamus also helps organize behavior related to survival: fighting, feeding, and fleeing.

That is why children whose thalamus is affected by prenatal alcohol exposure often get a panicked look in their eyes when faced with a sudden change or threat, or overloaded with information. When parents describe the children as being "stubborn," they are recognizing, perhaps, that the child diagnosed with FAS does not learn from experience in the same way other children do. This is not willful behavior on the part of the child; rather, the connections between past instructions or experience and current behavior just don't exist.

Alcohol use in the third trimester—the final three months of pregnancy—causes damage to the cerebral cortex, the outer shell of the brain. In the normal MRI shown previously (Figure 1.2), the cortex is folded in upon itself, forming the *gyri* and *sulci,* or valleys and ridges, in the brain. This folding occurs in the third trimester, producing increased brain surface area. In general, the more brain surface present in the cortex, the higher the level of cognitive functioning.

When a woman uses alcohol during the third trimester, however, brain cell migration is disrupted, interfering with the development of the gyri and sulci and significantly reducing brain surface area. As seen in Figure 1.5, also an MRI of a child with FAS, the brain is small, there are very few folds in the cortex of the brain, and the surface of the brain is quite flat (known as *lisencephaly*). These changes may be among the major factors producing the global intellectual disability seen in many children with FAS.

LISENCEPHALY DUE TO HEAVY THIRD TRIMESTER EXPOSURE TO ALCOHOL

FIG 1.5

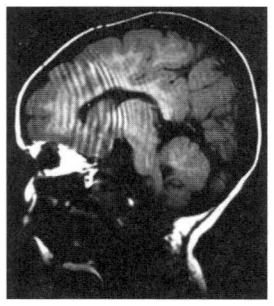

TERMINOLOGY

In the initial conceptualization of damage caused by prenatal alcohol exposure, if a woman drank alcohol during pregnancy and gave birth to a child who showed partial or no apparent expression of physical features characteristic of alcohol exposure, her child was said to have fetal alcohol effects (FAE). These children may have had minimal to moderate facial changes or no changes at all, but usually they had some problems with intellectual, behavioral, or emotional development. These difficulties were known to have an impact on learning and long-term development, though just how extensively FAE affected the child was less clear.

More recently, research has demonstrated that children with FAE may have significant structural and functional changes in the brain, even though they lack overt physical manifestation of the alcohol exposure. Guidelines published by the Institute of Medicine (IOM)[17] and the Centers for Disease Control and Prevention (CDC)[11] have attempted to lay out diagnostic criteria that can be applied to the varied pictures with which children prenatally exposed to alcohol can present. Based upon a comprehensive evaluation by a multidisciplinary team, children can be assigned an alcohol exposure-related diagnosis based on the following criteria:

- **Growth retardation**: current or past weight and/or height less than 10th percentile adjusted for age and gender.
- **Facial dysmorphology**: abnormal measurements of the upper lip (rank 4 or 5) *and* the philtrum (rank 4 or 5) *and* shortened palpebral fissures, according to analysis of facial features utilizing the *Lip-Philtrum Guide* and digital facial photograph based on the criteria of Astley and Clarren.[18,19]
- **Central nervous system abnormalities**: demonstration of structural, neurological, or functional CNS deficits[11] as documented by the presence of microcephaly (current head circumference below 10th percentile for age and gender) and/or functional deficits demonstrated as global cognitive delays with performance below the 3rd percentile on standardized testing or three or more domains of

neurodevelopmental functioning more than 2 standard deviations below the normed mean on standardized measures of neurocognitive, self-regulatory, or adaptive functioning.

Following these criteria, individuals who meet all physical criteria for growth impairment and facial dysmorphology as well as neurodevelopmental deficits receive a diagnosis of fetal alcohol syndrome (FAS). Individuals with confirmed prenatal alcohol exposure, facial dysmorphology, and neurodevelopmental deficits but with normal growth (height and weight) patterns, are diagnosed as partial FAS (*pFAS*). Individuals who have confirmed exposure and meet criteria for neurodevelopmental deficits but do not meet criteria for facial dysmorphology are classified as alcohol related neurodevelopmental disorder (*ARND*), and individuals with confirmed prenatal exposure and with malformations, including dysmorphic facial changes, but normal growth and normal neurodevelopment fall into the category of alcohol related birth defects (*ARBD*).

In April 2004, a group of federal agencies developed a consensus definition of fetal alcohol spectrum disorders (FASDs):

…an umbrella term describing the range of effects that can occur in an individual whose mother drank during pregnancy. These effects may include physical, mental, behavioral, and/or learning disabilities with possible lifelong implications.[20]

FASDs is not meant to serve as a diagnostic term, but rather a unifying one to help us appreciate the many ways in which prenatal alcohol exposure can become manifest in the affected individual. For our purposes, we will use the term "FASDs" throughout this book when the information applies to all alcohol-exposed children, including those with a diagnosis of FAS, pFAS, or ARND. When the information specifically refers to children with a specific diagnosis, such as FAS or ARND, we will use those terms. It is important to stress that FASDs is not a diagnostic term; it indicates only children affected by prenatal alcohol exposure and not a specific condition. This approach is consistent with the newly published DSM 5 mental health criteria for Neurodevelopmental Disorder with Prenatal Alcohol Exposure (ND-PAE).[21]

MISDIAGNOSIS AND MISSED DIAGNOSES

If diagnosis of alcohol-affected children were as easy as the terminology implies, we could move on from this discussion to other more important topics. But the truth is, there is great controversy as to how and when to diagnose children who may have been affected by their mother's use of alcohol during pregnancy. The key barrier to diagnosis is the lack of information regarding maternal alcohol use during pregnancy. Recent studies in general populations of pregnant women report that anywhere from 16% to 35% of the women have drunk some amount of alcohol during gestation, with the highest risk population frequently comprising middle class, well-educated women.[2] However, prenatal care providers often are reluctant to address their patients' drinking, and as a result alcohol use continues to lead to FASDs—one of the most commonly missed complications of pregnancy and early childhood.

Another difficulty in diagnosis relates to the lack of physical sequelae among the majority of alcohol-exposed children. Through the history of work with FAS, facial changes have been recognized as an essential component of diagnosis. In 2001, the researchers Susan Astley and Sterling Clarren evaluated the correlation of facial changes with brain dysfunction in a population of alcohol-exposed children.[18] The authors found that children with more severe facial changes demonstrated more severely impaired levels of cognitive, neuropsychological, and visual motor functioning. More recently, Astley emphasized the importance of the specificity of facial criteria in concluding a child has FAS.[15,22] At the same time, new research is demonstrating the primary role growth status (height and weight) has in recognizing children at risk from prenatal alcohol exposure.[7]

The clarification of these diagnostic issues is important for all those who care for children, especially children's health care providers whose role is to recognize those children who may be at risk from prenatal exposure to alcohol and foster and adoptive parents who must advocate for the child to ensure access to early intervention programs. Without a diagnosis of alcohol-related risk, many children and adolescents will not be deemed eligible for early intervention and school-based treatment programs, nor will insurance companies pay for related health care interventions. Parents and caregivers thus find themselves in a position of advocating for young people not deemed "sick enough" to receive services.

In October 2005, the Centers for Disease Control and Prevention (CDC) published guidelines for the identification and referral of persons with fetal alcohol syndrome.[11] The underlying goal of their report was to clarify the diagnosis of FAS, so as to enhance practicing clinicians' ability to recognize and refer patients who may have been negatively affected by prenatal alcohol exposure. However, for practicing clinicians, the CDC's guidelines contain many confusing features. The recommendation that substantial prenatal alcohol use must be confirmed runs counter to published data that document the impact of relatively small amounts of alcohol use in pregnancy; further, any thresholds for safe use have not been empirically validated, and as the authors of the CDC article acknowledge, it is extremely difficult to confirm prenatal alcohol use because denial, minimization, and inaccurate memories in birth parents are common.

These difficulties are documented by a study[23] currently underway at the Children's Research Triangle's children's mental health center. A wide variety of children and adolescents, key among them foster and adopted children, are referred for evaluation and treatment of behavioral, developmental, and mental health problems. An average of 200 children per year undergo a comprehensive medical, mental health, and neurodevelopmental assessment at the center, and about 600 children per year receive treatment services. Approximately 1/3 of the children evaluated each year receive a diagnosis within the fetal alcohol spectrum.

In assessing a sample of charts from the clinic, we found a significant difference in the diagnosis the children were referred with versus the diagnosis they received after a full evaluation by our multidisciplinary team. Of 51 children who came in to our clinic with a diagnosis related to prenatal alcohol exposure, only 31 actually met criteria for a diagnosis within FASDs. From the opposite perspective, of 156 children who after full assessment received a diagnosis within the fetal alcohol spectrum, only 31 (19.9%) had been referred to the clinic with a diagnosis related to prenatal alcohol exposure; 80.1% of children with FASDs had not been recognized. These data demonstrate the high rate of misdiagnosis and missed diagnoses related to FASDs. This has tremendous implications for treatment, including the use of medications to address behavioral difficulties. At the time of referral, 11 of the 156 children and youth with FASDs were on medications to treat ADHD. After assessment, ADHD medications were recommended to only one of these individuals. Twenty-two other children and youth with FASDs who had not presented on medications were prescribed ADHD medications following assessment. Appropriate use of medication is of vital importance in children with FASDs. Several research studies have pointed out that children with FASDs who also meet criteria for ADHD respond to medication therapy differently than children with ADHD who did not have a history of prenatal exposure to alcohol.[14,24]

These data point out the many ways in which the health and mental health care systems are failing children and adolescents affected by prenatal alcohol exposure. The American Academy of Pediatrics has recognized health care providers' failure to identify children affected by prenatal alcohol exposure and has formed a special academy committee, working with the Centers for Disease Control and Prevention to integrate FASDs screening and interventions into the academy's *Bright Futures*[25] protocols. These screening processes seek to focus on the functional neurobehavioral deficits found in children with FASDs rather than only on the facial and growth characteristics.

Once children with FASDs are recognized, there must be an immediate effort to obtain diagnostic and therapeutic services. Streissguth and colleagues have noted that early diagnosis, especially prior to the age of six years, coupled with earliest intervention is one of the strongest correlates with an improved outcome for the child long term.[26,27]

Delayed or incorrect diagnosis, especially among children who do not have the sentinel facial dsymorphology associated with FAS, may lead to a higher incidence of secondary disabilities[27,28] and greater need for special education services.

The role of the pediatrician and other children's health care providers is clear: early recognition of the child or youth with FASDs and referral to a provider who can conduct a full evaluation and develop a treatment plan that incorporates mental health treatment, behavioral management strategies, and special education services.[28]

UNDERSTANDING ADOLESCENTS WITH FASDs: THE CONCEPT OF BEHAVIORAL TERATOLOGY

This book focuses on adolescents affected by prenatal alcohol exposure. However, in reality, the young people under discussion often have multiple other factors impinging on their early and later social, emotional, academic and behavioral development. Vorhees in 1989[29] recognized a phenomenon he termed "behavioral teratology." There are three basic principles of behavioral teratology:

1. The impact of exposure to a foreign agent on the fetus's developing central nervous system and behavior is a function of multiple factors.
2. Damage to the central nervous system (brain) during the prenatal period has effects across the lifespan.
3. Central nervous system injury may result in behavioral impairments rather than physical birth defects.

With these three tenets in mind, I have built on the work of Vorhees, Linda Mayes, and others to develop a schematic representation of neurobehavioral teratology: the developmental progression of what we recognize as the picture of FASDs in the adolescent (Figure 1.6).

Beginning at the top of the graphic, it can be seen that in addition to prenatal exposure to alcohol or any other substance, there are other teratogenic exposures, such as lead, that can affect prenatal brain development. In addition, maternal factors such as education, poverty, living conditions, or even maternal stress can influence prenatal development. Postnatal influences, ranging from toxic elements in the environment (tobacco, marijuana, or methamphetamine smoke; lead in the painted walls of the home) to the abilities of the mother and the infant to read one another's cues and respond appropriately in their dance of early attunement, have an impact on early brain development, ultimately establishing developmental competency in the growing child.

A MODEL FOR NEUROBEVAVIORAL TERATOLOGY

FIG 1.6

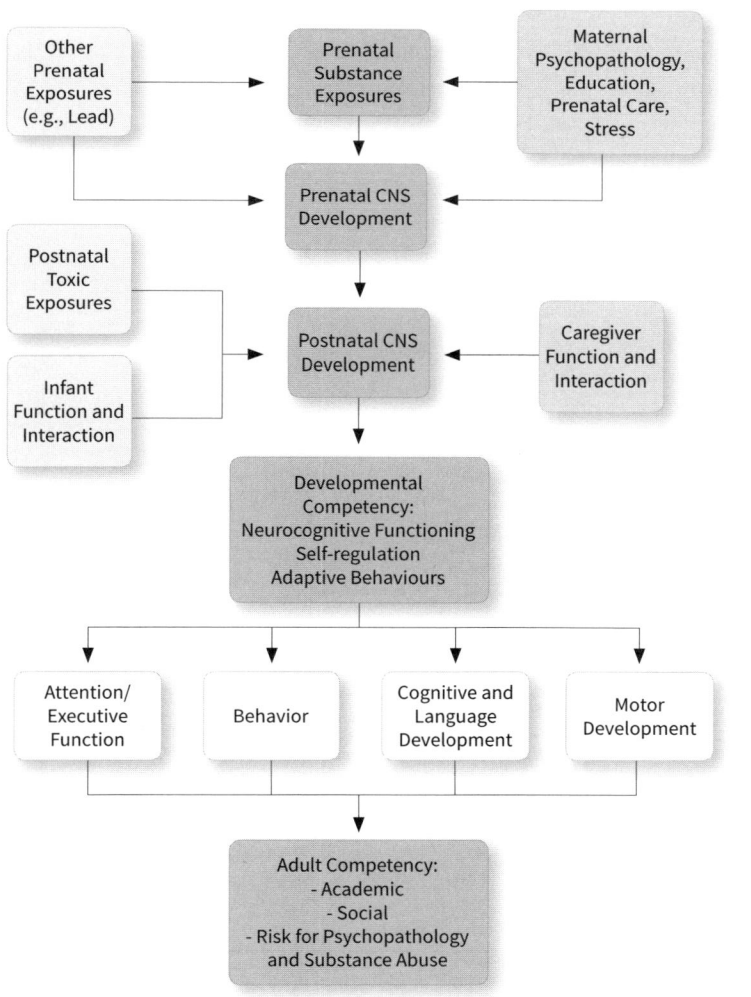

This base of developmental competency at a young age sets the stage for adult competency, measured from both an outcome and functional perspective.

What does all this mean? It means that children with prenatal alcohol exposure are born with biologically based developmental risk factors that can be influenced, for better or worse, by the environment in which the child and adolescent are raised. There may be limits to how well the child can do due to severity of damage induced by the alcohol exposure, but for each individual child those limits are unknown. It is up to parents and caregivers to advocate for their child, to insist on best care opportunities through the health care, mental health care, and educational systems, so that their child can reach his or her full potential.

NOTES

1. May PA, Gossage JP, Kalberg WO, Robinson LK, Buckley D, Manning M, Hoyme HE. Prevalence and epidemiologic characteristics of FASD from various research methods with an emphasis on recent in-school studies. *Dev Disabil Res Rev.* 2009;15(3):176-92.

2. Chasnoff IJ, Wells AM. FASD in Primary Prenatal Care: Screening and Brief Intervention. Final report to the Maternal and Child Health Bureau, Health Resources and Services Administration, US Department of Health and Human Services. Washington DC; 2013.

3. 2008-2009 National Survey on Drug Use and Health. Substance Abuse and Mental Health Services Administration, https://nsduhweb.rti.org/, Accessed May 15, 2014.

4. Astley SJ, Olson HC, Kerns K, et al. Neuropsychological and behavioral outcomes from a comprehensive magnetic resonance study of children with fetal alcohol spectrum disorders. *Canadian Journal of Clinical Pharmacology.* 2009;16:e178–e201.

5. Carmichael Olson, H, Feldman JJ, Streissguth AP, Sampson PD, Bookstein FL. Neuropsychological deficits in adolescents with Fetal Alcohol Syndrome: clinical findings. *Alcoholism: Clinical & Experimental Research.* 1998;22(9):1998–2012

6. Carmichael Olson H, Streissguth AP, Sampson, PD, Barr HM, Bookstein, FL, Thiede, K. Association of prenatal alcohol exposure with behavioral and learning problems in early adolescence. *Journal of the American Academy of Child and Adolescent Psychiatry.* 1997;36(9):1187–1194.

7. Chasnoff IJ, Wells AM, Telford E, Schmidt C, Messer G. Neurodevelopmental functioning in children with FAS, pFAS, and ARND *Journal of Developmental and Behavioral Pediatrics.* 2010; in press.

8. Coles CD, Brown RT, Smith IE, Platzman KA, Erickson S, Falek A. Effects of prenatal alcohol exposure at school age: I. Physical and cognitive development. *Neurotoxicology and Teratology.* 1991;13:357–367.

9. Jones K, Smith DW. Recognition of the fetal alcohol syndrome in early infancy. *Lancet.* 1973;ii:999-1201.

10   Disney ER, Iacono W, McGue M, Tully E, Legrand L. Strengthening the case: prenatal alcohol exposure is associated with increased risk for conduct disorder. Pediatrics. 2008;122; e1225–e1230. doi:10.1542/peds. 2008–1380.

11   Sarkola T, Gissler M, Kahila H, Autti-Rämö I, Halmesmäki E. Alcohol and substance abuse identified during pregnancy: maternal morbidity, child morbidity and welfare interventions. *Acta Paediatrica* 2012; 101:784-90.

12   Chasnoff I.J. *The Mystery of Risk: Drugs, Alcohol, Pregnancy, and the Vulnerable Child.* NTI Publishing: Chicago, Illinois, 2011.

13   Kodituwakku, P.W. Defining the behavioral phenotype in children with fetal alcohol spectrum disorders: A review. *Neuroscience and Biobehavioral Reviews.* 2007;31:192–201.

14   Coles CD, Platzman KA, Rakind-Hood CL, Brown RT, Falek A, Smith IE. A comparison of children affected by prenatal alcohol exposure and attention deficit, hyperactivity disorder. *Alcoholism: Clinical and Experimental Research.* 1997;21:150-161.

15   Astley SJ, Aylward EH, Olson HC, et al. Magnetic resonance imaging outcomes from a comprehensive magnetic resonance study of children with fetal alcohol spectrum disorders. *Alcoholism: Clinical and Experimental Research.* 2009;33:1671-1689.

16   Jacobson S, Jacobson J, Sokol RJ, Martier S. and Ager J. Prenatal alcohol exposure and infant information processing ability. *Child Development.* 1993;64:1706–1721.

17   Stratton K, Howe C, Battaglia F. *Fetal Alcohol Syndrome: Diagnosis, Epidemiology, Prevention, and Treatment.* Washington, DC: National Academy Press. Institute of Medicine; 1996.

18   Astley SJ, Clarren SK. Measuring the facial phenotype of individuals with prenatal alcohol exposure: correlations with brain dysfunction. *Alcohol & Alcoholism.* 2001;36:147-159.

19   Astley SJ, Clarren SK. Diagnosing the full spectrum of fetal alcohol-exposed individuals: introducing the 4-digit diagnostic code. *Alcohol & Alcoholism.* 2000;35:400-412.

20   Bertrand J, Floyd RL, Weber MK, et al. National Task Force on FAS/FAE. Fetal Alcohol Syndrome: Guidelines for Referral and Diagnosis; 2004; Atlanta, GA: Centers for Disease Control and Prevention.

21 American Psychiatric Association. *Diagnostic and Statistical Manual of Mental Disorders, 5th Edition: DSM-5.* Arlington, VA: American Psychiatric Publishing, 2013.

22 Astley SJ. Comparison of the 4-digit diagnostic code and the Hoyme diagnostic guidelines for Fetal Alcohol Spectrum Disorders. *Pediatrics.* 2006;118:1532-1545.

23 Chasnoff IJ, Wells AM, King L. Misdiagnosis and missed diagnoses in children affected by prenatal exposure to alcohol. Manuscript submitted for publication, 2014.

24 Oesterheld JR, Kofoed L, Tervo R, Fogas B, Wilson A, Fiechtner H. Effectiveness of methyplphenidate in Native American children with fetal alcohol syndrome and attention deficit/hyperactivity disorder: A controlled pilot study. *Journal of Child and Adolescent Psychopharmacology.* 1998;8:39-48.

25 Bright Futures. http://brightfutures.aap.org/

26 Streissguth AP, Barr HM, Kogan J, Bookstein FL. *Understanding the occurrence of secondary disabilities in clients with fetal alcohol syndrome (FAS) and fetal alcohol effects (FAE).* Final report to the Centers for Disease Control and Prevention. Seattle: University of Washington, Fetal Alcohol and Drug Unit, 1996.

27 Streissguth AP, Bookstein FL, Barr HM, Sampson PD, O'Malley K, Young JK. Risk factors for adverse life outcomes in fetal alcohol syndrome and fetal alcohol effects. *J Dev Behav Pediatr.* 2004;25:228-238.

28 Autti-Ramo I. Twleve-year follow-up of children exposed to alcohol in utero. *Dev Med Child Neurol.* 2000;42:406-411.

29 Vorhees CV. Concepts in teratology and developmental toxicology derived from animal research. *Ann NY ACAD Sci.* 1989;562:31-41.

CHAPTER 2 · *Psychology*

FETAL ALCOHOL SPECTRUM DISORDERS IN THE TEENAGE YEARS

Julie Kable, Ph.D.

Dr. Julie Kable, Assistant Professor of Psychiatry at Emory University School of Medicine, looks at how those who have been affected by prenatal exposure to alcohol manage through the teenage years. In the best of circumstances, this period of adolescence is often challenging for both the teenager and the parents, and even more so for the teenager affected by prenatal exposure to alcohol. Dr. Kable offers insight on emotional, learning, and identity issues. As she states, "Unfortunately, the teen years may result in the greatest observable impact of prenatal alcohol exposure on the brain."

The teen years are a period of rapid physical changes. Teens are faced with increased demands for self-governance, and they strive for greater independence. This period of transition between childhood and adulthood is often portrayed as being full of turmoil[1] even for typically developing teens and their families. By its completion, the teen is expected to transition into being a responsible and productive adult member of society. To assist with the transition, the teen develops an increased interest in peers or social groups. Parental guidance and supervision in decision-making becomes less desired. This transition in roles within the family can be stressful. Even typically developing teens stumble and encounter difficulties as they learn to deal with new conflicts, pressures, and opportunities. The outcomes of this stage of development often have lifetime ramifications as the teen reaches sexual maturity, works to develop a sense of self-identity, and begins to pursue a career direction. Parents often have great concern about their teen's ability to handle these new challenges.

Just as individuals with Fetal Alcohol Spectrum Disorders (FASDs) often struggle as an infant with learning to walk, they frequently have additional difficulties learning to handle the new roles and responsibilities that the teen years bring. For parents of a teen with FASDs, this stage of development can be incredibly anxiety provoking; protecting a teen is often much more complicated than preventing an infant from hurting himself while learning to walk.

From a developmental perspective, the teen years are associated with increased myelination of portions of the brain involved in inhibitory control and decision-making.[2,3] This leads to progressive improvements in regulating emotions. In addition, the ability to see multiple facets of a problem develops. Complex decision-making becomes possible. These changes, however, may not manifest until young adulthood. This is because areas of the brain involved in inhibitory control and decision-making continue their growth beyond the teen years.

Often the gap between individuals with FASDs and their typically developing peers seems at its greatest during this stage of development. Unfortunately, the teen years may result in the greatest observable impact of prenatal alcohol exposure on the brain. This is because the areas of the brain that are crucial to successful functioning in the teen years are damaged by prenatal alcohol. The combination of poor impulse control, difficulties with inhibiting responses, and an increased emotional reactivity, all dependent on brain maturation, has been linked to poor outcomes.[3]

Research over a 40-year period has documented the nature of these deficits. Neuroimaging suggests that the cognitive and behavioral impairments seen in individuals with FASDs are linked to specific areas of the brain impacted by prenatal alcohol exposure, including malformations and reductions in the size of the whole brain and specific areas of the brain. Functional neuroimaging studies have documented how the brain works in individuals with FASDs. Research has found that the pattern of brain activation while performing cognitive tasks is different if there is a history of prenatal alcohol exposure. This suggests that the brain works differently in a teen with FASDs. Finally, it has been found that the ability of the neurons to efficiently communicate with each other can be damaged by prenatal alcohol exposure. These physical alterations in the brain of teens with FASDs result in impairments in cognitive and behavioral functioning.

The first of the areas of altered impairment is in *neurocognitive or learning* skills. The second area of deficit is *behavioral regulation.* This involves the regulation of attention and arousal or emotions. Finally, the ability to function within one's environment or *adaptive living skills* has been found to be impaired. Each of these areas of deficit has important implications for the challenges with which a teen with FASDs has to cope.

NEUROCOGNITIVE IMPAIRMENTS

Individuals with FASDs may have lower intelligence, difficulty with abstract reasoning, and problems applying knowledge to new situations. Impairments in intellectual functioning are commonly seen in children with FASDs, but the majority does not meet criteria for "intellectual disability." The average level of intellectual functioning as measured by a standard intelligence quotient (IQ) has been estimated to be in the 70s. This level is often labeled the *Borderline range* of intellectual functioning. IQ scores in this range do not automatically result in services.

The range of IQs found in individuals with FASDs has been quite broad.[4] For those who meet criteria for an intellectual disability, a host of intervention services are available to support the individual. Unfortunately for those who do not meet criteria, this is not the case. Often the impairments in their cognitive functioning are not identified or treated. This leads to problems with basic life skills and planning, poor school achievement, and problems in job functioning.

Executive functioning skills refer to higher-order thinking processes needed to plan and organize responses and efforts to achieve goals.[5] These skills are often impaired in individuals with FASDs,[6,7] many of whom have been found to have difficulties mentally manipulating information. This is expressed when doing math problems or when asked to rotate or move something mentally. Thinking about steps involved in completing a task or other sequential information can be challenging. Children and youth with FASDs also struggle with changing strategies or thinking about things in more than one way, including applying knowledge to new situations. Transitioning from one activity to another sometimes can result in frustration. Repeatedly making the same mistakes as they struggle with incorporating new feedback into their responses is also symptomatic of executive skill deficits. Executive functioning skills are greatly influenced by maturation of the prefrontal cortex, in the anterior part of the brain, which has been found to be affected by prenatal alcohol.[8]

Teens with FASDs often have lower school achievement than expected. One of the well-documented areas of school deficit is in math functioning.[6] Specific damage from the prenatal alcohol exposure has been found to cause damage to areas of the brain involved in learning math.[9,10] Several negative school-related outcomes, including repeating grades, school failure, and dropping out of school also have been linked to prenatal alcohol exposure.[11,12] Many things influence these outcomes. The teen's developmental status and emotional functioning are two very important factors. The teen's community and family support for academic success also is an important influence. Individuals with FASDs need frequent monitoring of their academic progress. This should be done through standardized testing and reports from teachers regarding the teen's classroom performance. By providing appropriate help when needed, these adverse academic outcomes hopefully can be avoided.

Individuals with FASDs often have memory problems.[13] These difficulties with memory can be expressed in a wide variety of ways and through everyday behaviors. Often the children and youth have difficulty recalling recently learned information or have problems with retrieving information. This can be very frustrating to parents, teachers, and work supervisors. The poor recall is often misinterpreted as "bad behavior" or as "laziness." Often the adult will report that the teen could do it one day but not the next, so it must be that the teen does not want to do it. In fact, this memory impairment is the result of the impact of prenatal alcohol on portions of the brain involved in memory storage and retrieval.[14] Often the teen will need frequent reminders to successfully complete tasks. These memory impairments often result in teens' losing or misplacing possessions and contribute to their problems solving complex problems.

A specific area of memory functioning that appears to be impacted by prenatal alcohol exposure is known as *working memory*. Working memory involves using a "mental sketchpad." The mental sketchpad is used to analyze information. A common example of this skill is to ask someone to recite her or his telephone number backwards. To do this, a person has to use working memory. Some researchers[15] have concluded that problems in managing goals in working memory are responsible for much of the cognitive impairment seen in individuals with FASDs.

Another area often impaired in individuals with FASDs is their ability to perceive and analyze visual or spatial information.[6] They may have disorganized or poorly planned drawings or constructions. This may result in everyday problems understanding physical directions. Individuals with this type of problem also have difficulty solving puzzles or reading and following a map.

SELF-REGULATION

The ability to regulate one's attention and overall arousal level is an integral skill needed to acquire knowledge and to learn from one's experiences. We know that this basic interactive regulation is disrupted in infancy, often leading to a lifetime of difficulties with self-regulation skills.[13] Arousal problems initially are seen in the area of sleep problems in infancy. Infants with FASDs may have problems with going to sleep and also may have problems with staying asleep throughout the night or being easily awakened.[16,17] Sleep habits frequently are disrupted in typically developing teens, and these normal disruptions can make an affected individual's pre-existing sleep problems even worse. Maintaining and supporting positive sleep habits are important for helping an individual with FASDs' self-regulation skills.

Attention problems are commonly reported in individuals affected by prenatal alcohol exposure.[6] Many individuals with FASDs are diagnosed with an attention deficit disorder (ADD). There is concern that the ADD medications are not as helpful for individuals with FASDs and that the nature of the attention problems is slightly different[18] from that in individuals with ADD who were not prenatally exposed to alcohol. Children and youth with FASDs often have difficulties staying focused and struggle to sustain their mental effort. They also have problems with learning new things and shifting attention to focus on new things. They often are impulsive and/or disinhibited. In addition, many have difficulties with waiting for things, complying with rules, and delaying gratification. Deficits in this area can result in problems with confabulating, taking others' possessions, and engaging in risky behaviors.

Children and youth affected by prenatal alcohol exposure frequently have been found to have behavioral outbursts and difficulty calming down from the outburst. They often are described as moody or irritable. Their poor emotional control and instability can be aggravating to those around them. Parents report that their children seem to have very little control over their behavior during these episodes. The term *affective storm* or *emotional storm* seems to best describe the event. Once the storm has blown over, the individual may well regret his behavior and apologize. Individuals with FASDs also tend to be easily overwhelmed or over stimulated. They struggle with handling exciting events, like parties or holidays. In the normal life of the teen years, there are many anxiety-provoking events so that this problem may feel more intense relative to earlier stages of development. The physical size of the teen may also result in the parents' not feeling safe during one of these episodes. Some parents have even sought assistance from law enforcement to protect themselves, the teen, and other family members.

Individuals with FASDs often are described as being hyper-responsive to events around them and may have difficulty adapting to change.[15,19] These children and youth often easily give up or get frustrated, particularly when given negative feedback.[20] A teen with FASDs once left school as a result of frustration about his learning experiences. The school called the police out of concern for the teen. When the police officer found the teen, the teen became highly excited and grabbed for the officer's gun. Fortunately, this incident did not result in any harm to the teen or the officer. Clearly, however, there was great potential for harm in this situation. It is important to avoid over exciting a teen with FASDs. Getting too excited results in the teens not being able to effectively use the problem-solving portions of her brain. Often the best approach is to try first to calm the teen and then approach her and begin to help her problem-solve the dilemma. Some parents of teens with FASDs have provided educational trainings to their local law enforcement officials to prevent such disasters from happening to their teen with FASDs.

A great deal of research has been conducted regarding the negative impact of prenatal alcohol on the brain circuitry involved in regulating attention and arousal or emotions.[21-39] This research suggests that the problems in this area have a clear basis in early brain development. Early signs of dysregulation are manifest as increased stress reactions[40-42] and increased levels of negative emotions.[43] Later, these problems result in the young person's being given psychiatric diagnoses,[29,44-49] having increased problems with substance abuse,[50-52] and having increased legal difficulties.[53,54] These problems result from a combination of alcohol-related brain damage and adverse environmental circumstance often encountered by individuals with FASDs. Children and youth with FASDs often have a history of involvement with child protective services. They often may have been born to families with limited resources and may have had multiple primary caregivers over their lifespan. Each of these factors adds an additional layer of risk factors for adverse outcomes.

Many other developmental disorders manifest themselves as problems with attention and arousal. Understanding the fundamental differences for these disorders relative to FASDs is important for knowing how to improve learning. The table depicts the arousal dysregulation problems of individuals with FASDs as compared to other common psychiatric disorders. Specifically, it compares children with autism and attention deficit hyperactivity disorder (ADHD) and includes information regarding the impact of prenatal cocaine exposure on arousal. The arousal dysfunction is discussed in terms of what is needed to achieve *homeostasis* for the individual, i.e., achieving an optimal balance in arousal level needed to improve learning.

The following table depicts the arousal dysregulation problems of children with FASDs as compared to other common psychiatric disorders (Autism and ADHD) and to the impact of prenatal cocaine exposure. The dysfunction is discussed in terms of what is needed to achieve homeostasis for the individual and what environmental changes help improve learning.

DIFFERENTIATING NEURODEVELOPMENTAL DISORDER IN CHILDREN WITH PRENATAL ALCOHOL EXPOSURE FROM OTHER DEVELOPMENTAL DISORDERS

TABLE

DISORDER	DYSFUNCTION	DIFFERENCES	STIMULUS CHANGES NEEDED
AUTISM	Easily over aroused	Downward shift in need for central stimulation or reduced ability to modulate or habituate stimulus input	Reduce sensory input
ADHD	Under aroused	Shift in level of central stimulation found to be optimal from inadequate neuro-transmission of incoming stimulation	Respond to stimulant medications and increases in arousal
FASD	Arousal dysfunction	Slower gating of incoming stimulation and reduced capacity to inhibit attending to distracting stimuli	Respond to simplification of sensory input (fewer distracters and slower presentation)
COCAINE EXPOSURE	Heightened arousal responses	Over aroused by stimulation and difficulties returning to baseline levels. Also has difficulties with maintaining inhibitory control	Monitoring of arousal level so stimulus input can be modified when too high. Longer periods allowed for recovery of functioning

Individuals with autism often are easily over-aroused. They need to reduce sensory input to improve their learning. This is the result of a downward shift in their need for stimulation and a reduced ability to modulate or habituate to things in the environment. In contrast, children with an attention deficit disorder (ADD) are often better described as being chronically under-aroused. They require increases in arousal to improve learning. This can be achieved by the use of stimulant medications or by increasing the arousal level of the learning material. For example, individuals with ADD can often maintain very effective attentional skills when playing a stimulating videogame. In contrast, they often struggle performing in a traditional classroom.

Individuals with FASDs are best described as having arousal dysfunction. Their problems result from their slower ability to gate incoming stimulation and a reduced capacity to block out other distracting events. To assist with improving learning, individuals with FASDs benefit most from simplifying their sensory input. This means having fewer distracters and slowing the pace of the instruction to improve learning skills.[55]

Some individuals with FASDs may also have damage to their attention and arousal regulation skills from other sources. They may have inherited genes that disrupt brain development. In addition, many individuals with FASDs have other prenatal exposures (i.e. cocaine exposure). Research on children with a history of cocaine exposure suggests that this prenatal exposure is associated with heightened arousal responses to stressors. Children prenatally exposed to cocaine also have problems with returning to normal levels after the stressor is gone. Their arousal responses, however, are completely normal in the absence of a stressor. Understanding a teen's specific abilities to regulate his attention and arousal will help teachers and parents know how to improve the young person's learning skills.

ADAPTIVE PROBLEMS

There are four domains of adaptive functioning that have been commonly studied: communication, independent living skills, social skills, and motor skills. Individuals with FASDs have been found to have impairment in each of these areas. Adaptive communication refers to understanding and expressing oneself in the everyday environment. Impairment often seen in young children with FASDs includes initial difficulty learning a language; in the teen years, the symptoms are more likely to impact the pragmatic use of language.[56,57] Pragmatic use of language refers to using language to effectively communicate a message in everyday life. Impairment in this area limits the young person's ability to communicate her needs to others and using language so that the listener understands. She also will struggle with comprehending the meaning of communications from others. There may be problems linking words with feelings and understanding jokes or metaphors. They also have problems with making comments that seem out of context. Their family and peers complain that the young person talks too much or does not know when to stop talking.

Attainment of appropriate skills to function on one's own is vital for establishing independence. Individuals with FASDs often have early impairments in basic life skills, such as dressing, toileting, and making change.[19] Although these deficits may have resolved by the teen years, teens with FASDs face additional challenges associated with taking care of their basic needs. For example, problems with personal hygiene may persist into the teen years. Often individuals with FASDs have a poor understanding of the rules of personal safety,[58] which may result in the teen's placing himself in harm's way.

Finally, young people with prenatal alcohol exposure often struggle with learning to perceive time spans appropriately and with organizing daily schedules.[59] This leads to problems with managing daily activities and keeping appointments. Further adaptive deficits may impact their ability to manage finances and secure and/or maintain employment.

Impairment in social skills also is commonly reported in individuals with FASDs.[60] The symptoms are different from other developmental disorders, such as autism, which are known to impact social skills. In fact, individuals with FASDs often are overly friendly with strangers but have difficulty reading social cues. They struggle with understanding social consequences and using social problem-solving skills. Deficits in this area often lead to individuals with FASDs being characterized as gullible or naïve and being unaware of the effects of their actions on others. They are often described as being immature or acting too young. They often have difficulty making and keeping friends. Parents express concern that the youth use poor judgment in choosing friends, their friendships often being described as superficial. They often struggle with understanding personal space and making inappropriate social overtures. Of even greater concern, young people affected by prenatal alcohol exposure are easily led by others. In the teen years, this can result in the teen finding himself in a great deal of trouble at school and with the legal system.

Impairments in motor functioning have been identified throughout the lifespan of individuals with FASDs. Motor skill deficits are most noticeable in the first five years of life[61] but later impairment in motor skills also has been documented.[4,62-64] Specific areas of motor deficits include fine motor strength and coordination[65,66] and increased motor tremors.[67,68] Impairment in balance,[68,69] motor clumsiness,[70] and gait abnormalities[68,71] also have been reported. These deficits have important implications for job placement and should be appropriately evaluated to assist with education and career planning.

MALADAPTIVE BEHAVIORS AND HOW TO PREVENT THEM

The combination of the various deficits previously discussed often leads to maladaptive behaviors. Parents of teens with FASDs have recounted numerous stories of risky and potentially life-threatening behaviors. Parents also commonly report unusual or illogical behaviors that leave them scratching their heads. Advancements in technology have resulted in a host of new complaints from parents. Ordering an excessive number of movies from pay-per-view channels is a common complaint. Some report their child ordering additional movies even before the first one is completed, suggesting the teen was not really even watching the movies. Losing or inappropriately using cell phones is another (see chapter 8) common complaint. Inappropriate ordering from on-line websites occurs with some frequency. This is thanks to computers that automatically log you on to accounts.

To make matters worse, the behavioral expectations of the adults and systems within which adolescents interact become less tolerant as the young person grows older. Numerous families raising a child with FASDs have had to face a teacher or school staff member telling them that "Now that your child is in middle/high school, we can no longer…." Often the on-going supports provided by the schools are vital to maintaining the teen's successful functioning. When appropriate supports are removed and the individual does not have sufficient capacity to cope, the individual often engages in maladaptive behaviors. Without appropriate supervision and assistance with problem-solving and dealing with the various societal pressures placed upon them, teens with FASDs will often make bad or illogical choices. To prevent these outcomes, it is important to use gradual transitions when removing supports and supervision and to evaluate the adolescent's success with each transition or change.

The chronological age of the teen with FASDs should not be used to determine whether or not she is ready for a new responsibility. Instead, age should be used to trigger an evaluation of her readiness for graduated responsibilities and an analysis of her specific strengths as well as skill deficits. What needs to be taught to the individual before she can assume a specific responsibility also needs to be assessed. For example, attaining an age of 12 or 13 does not mean that the individual is ready to stay at home alone. Also, because she is now 16 does not mean she should have a driver's license. There is considerable variability in teens with FASDs so it is impossible to specify an age for a given milestone. Often professional consultation will be needed to assist the parent in completing this assessment and appropriately preparing the teen with sufficient skills and coping strategies to assume the responsibility.

Teenagers with FASDs often have completely normal facial features and body build. The lack of physical cues impedes others' realization that the young person may need accommodations or that developmental expectations should change. Often, conversations with the teen may leave a false impression of the teen's competence. Advocacy and communication with other adults who interact with the teen may be needed. This will ensure that appropriate supports are put into place to minimize maladaptive responses.

GOAL ATTAINMENT PROBLEMS

One of the common pet peeves of parents of a teen with FASDs is that the young person cannot appropriately define a goal, work towards it, and ultimately achieve the goal. This is of concern to most parents because they intuitively know that this skill is vital for their teen's independence and life success. A teen will often decide he wants to do something but then change his mind. Although this occurs among typically developing teens, the frequency and short duration between the switches seems greater in teens with FASDs. Alternatively, many of the young people do not seem to be able to follow through with the necessary activities that will allow them to be successful. Deficits in this area are related to the poor executive functioning skills and problems with self-regulation or behavioral control. It is understandable that parents become frustrated, but unfortunately this will only cause further deterioration in the parent-teen relationship.

The teen might need help with understanding the steps or sequence of events that will lead to his or her desired outcome. This may involve several discussions. Visually showing the steps may be necessary to assist her in understanding. The work effort needed and potential barriers that would need to be overcome must be discussed. The teen should be allowed to reevaluate his or her commitment to the goal based on this assessment. Negative feedback to the teen may lead to adverse outcomes as a result of his poor emotional control. Negative feedback may also interfere with his ability to take in or process the information needed to plan and carry out the steps needed to achieve the goal. Parents need considerable patience to be able to assist the teen through this process. Professional consultation may be needed for some decision-making to minimize parent–teen conflict.

BODILY CHANGES

The dramatic physical changes associated with adolescence can be mysterious and confusing for typically developing teens. When puberty starts, suddenly hair grows places where it has never been. Personal hygiene takes on a heightened level of concern as bodies begin to emit odors never before experienced. Females experience menstruation for the first time and have to learn many new skills to cope with this body change. When their breasts begin to develop, new demands are placed on them in their daily dressing routine. Males often experience changes in their vocalizations that are often the subject of gentle teasing to outright ridicule. Teens begin to have novel sensations and responses from their genitals. To cope with these massive changes, parents often attempt to have discussions to explain the metamorphosis. Pediatricians and other healthcare professionals provide educational materials to ease individuals through the changes. School systems attempt to provide anticipatory guidance by using videos often shown in same-sex classrooms. These efforts are commonly used with typically developing preteens and teens to assist them in preparing themselves for what to expect.

Unfortunately, for a teen with FASDs the training process is often more complicated and time consuming as a result of learning difficulties. For example, in tracking menstrual cycles, teens with FASDs are not in tune with their bodily cues or changes, and these girls with poor organization skills and time perception will find this skill more difficult. Often, as a result, females with FASDs may struggle with predicting the onset of menses. This can result in the need for an emergency change of clothing. Additional training in tracking the menstrual flow onset may be needed, including direct instruction on how to use a calendar. For some, positive behavioral supports to assist them with completing the calendar tracking may be needed. In addition, more extensive discussion of the bodily cues associated with onset may need to be held on repeated occasions to assist them with recognition. These talks may precede anticipated onset and also follow to retrospectively discuss what was different for them. The parent may need to keep a log of symptoms from month to month to assist the female adolescent with predicting onset and understanding her bodily cues.

Additional supports and discussions will often be needed to help a teen with FASDs in dealing with their sexuality. Although these discussions can be uncomfortable, it is important for the parent to persevere. The teen with FASDs needs to understand how to protect her or himself from disease and how to prevent an unwanted pregnancy. A parent should anticipate that this will require more than one conversation. The parent also should be aware that increased supervision might be needed until the young person is prepared to handle these responsibilities on his or her own.

PEER INFLUENCES

The term peer pressure is often associated with maladaptive behaviors. However, peer pressure also works to help maintain prosocial behavior. The developmental problems that teens with FASDs have contribute to their difficulties with understanding their social interactions and relationships. This makes it difficult for them to develop good quality peer relationships. As a result, the positive or prosocial peer influences can be absent.

The self-regulation problems also lead to problems with being able to function independently. When younger, parents complain the child cannot play by himself. As a teen, poor social skills often lead to frequent social isolation. Often to avoid the social isolation, the teen will seek out maladaptive peer interactions. Poor impulse control and difficulties with evaluating a situation can make the teen with FASDs vulnerable to exploitation. These young people need to have explicit instruction in social skills to assist in building positive peer relationships. Ongoing assistance or guidance in social problem-solving may also be needed to help them in negotiating complex peer interactions. Increased supervision during social interactions and efforts to facilitate structured social encounters may be required to assist the teen with learning appropriate social interactions skills.

Increased supervision of the various methods of social media communication is crucial. Even typically developing teens are finding this new frontier of social communication to be problematic. The increased supervision that is required, relative to supervision provided to their peers, can be a source of conflict at a time when teens want increased independence. Parents should keep in mind that research has shown that increased supervision of a teen acts as a buffer to prevent delinquency.[72] Consultation with a professional who has experience working with teens that have FASDs may aid in reducing family conflict around these competing interests.

PARENT FATIGUE

For many parents, the teen years can bring some relief in that the normally developing teen can be independent and helpful to the household. A parent may no longer need a babysitter as the teen can now stay at home alone or can provide free babysitting for younger children. A parent may also be able to delegate a responsibility to the teen, which can ease the parent's burden. Teens with a driver's license can run errands. They can pick up another child from practice or piano lessons or stop by the grocery store for something needed for the evening meal. These benefits can help outweigh the parental anxiety associated with their teen's assuming the new responsibilities. Unfortunately, for a parent of a teen with FASDs, these benefits are sparse or even non-existent.

Often the parents of a teen with FASDs have had to assume an expanded role, leading to fatigue. The lack of progress in their teen's skills can trigger anxiety about the future as well. The resistance from society to continue to provide the appropriate supports needed also adds an increased burden to caregiving. Parental fatigue and burn out accelerate. In the worst of circumstances, parents of a teen with FASDs have found themselves faced with having to seek assistance from law enforcement or making decisions about inpatient psychiatric care. Disruptions in placements have occurred for teens with FASDs because of parental burnout.

Parents have to work hard to make sure that they are taking care of themselves. They need appropriate supports and respite periods to maintain sufficient energy and resources to cope with the burdens of caregiving. Parental support groups for families parenting a child with FASDs may also be helpful and are available in some communities. Seeking professional consultation should not be viewed as a weakness but a necessity to cope with the burdens associated with parenting a teen with FASDs.

NOTES

1. Casey BJ, Jones RM, Levita L, Libby V, Pattwell SS, Ruberry EJ,... Somerville LH. The storm and stress of adolescence: insights from human imaging and mouse genetics. *Dev Psychobiol.,* 2010;52(3):225-235. doi: 10.1002/dev.20447.

2. Casey BJ, & Jones RM. Neurobiology of the adolescent brain and behavior: implications for substance use disorders. *J Am Acad Child Adolesc Psychiatry,* 2010;49(12):1189-1201; quiz 1285. doi: 10.1016/j.jaac.2010.08.017.

3. Casey BJ, Jones RM, & Hare TA. The adolescent brain. *Ann N Y Acad Sci,* 2008;1124:111-126. doi: 10.1196/annals.1440.010.

4. Mattson SN, Riley EP. A review of the neurobehavioral deficits in children with fetal alcohol syndrome or prenatal exposure to alcohol. *Alcohol Clin Exp Res,* 1998;22(2):279-294.

5. Lyon GR. The need for conceptual and theoretical clarity in the study of attention, memory, and executive funcitoning. In G. R. Lyon & N. A. Krasnegor (Eds.), *Attention, memory, and executive functioning* (pp. 3-10). Baltimore: Paul Brookes Publishing Co., 1996.

6. Kable JA, & Coles CD. Teratology of Alcohol: Implications for School Settings. In R. T. Brown (Ed.), *Handbook of Pediatric Psychology in School Settings.* Mahwah, NJ: Lawrence Erbaum Associates, 2004.

7. Mattson SN, Roesch SC, Fagerlund A, Autti-Ramo I, Lyons KL, May PA, ... Riley EP. Toward a neurobehavioral profile of fetal alcohol spectrum. *Alcoholism: Clinical & Experimental Research,* 2010;34(9):1640-1650.

8. Lebel C, Roussotte F, Sowell ER. Imaging the impact of prenatal alcohol exposure on the structure of the developing human brain. *Neuropsychology Review,* 2011;21(2), 102-118. doi: 10.1007/s11065-011-9163-0.

9. Lebel C, Rasmussen C, Wyper K, Andrew G, Beaulieu C. Brain microstructure is related to math ability in children with fetal alcohol spectrum disorder. *Alcohol Clin Exp Res,* 2010;34(2), 354-363. doi: ACER1097 [pii] 10.1111/j.1530-0277.2009.01097.x.

10. Riikonen R, Salonen I, Partanen K, Verho S. Brain perfusion SPECT and MRI in fetal alcohol syndrome. *Dev Med Child Neurol,* 1999;41(10):652-659.

11   Autti-Ramo I. Twelve-year follow-up of children exposed to alcohol in utero. *Dev Med Child Neurol,* 2000; 42(6):406-411.

12   Streissguth AP, Barr HM, Kogan, J, Bookstein, FL. *Understanding the occurrence of secondary disabilities in clients with fetal alcohol syndrome (FAS) and Fetal Alcohol Effects (FAE). Final Report.* Seattle, WA: University of Seattle Washington Publication Service., 1996.

13   Kable JA, Coles CD. The impact of prenatal alcohol exposure on neurophysiological encoding of environmental events at six months. *Alcohol Clin Exp Res,* 2004;28(3):489-496. doi: 00000374-200403000-00016 [pii].

14   Coles CD, Goldstein FC, Lynch ME, Chen X, Kable JA, Johnson KC, Hu, X. Memory and brain volume in adults prenatally exposed to alcohol. *Brain and Cognition,* 2011;75(1), 67-77. doi: 10.1016/j.bandc.2010.08.013.

15   Kodituwakku PW, Handmaker NS, Cutler SK, Weathersby EK, Handmaker SD. Specific impairments in self-regulation in children exposed to alcohol prenatally. *Alcohol Clin Exp Res,* 1995;19(6):1558-1564.

16   Pesonen AK, Raikkonen K, Matthews K, Heinonen K, Paavonen JE, Lahti, J., . . . Strandberg, T. Prenatal origins of poor sleep in children. *Sleep,* 2009;32(8):1086-1092.

17   Scher MS, Richardson GA, Coble PA, Day NL, Stoffer DS. The effects of prenatal alcohol and marijuana exposure: disturbances in neonatal sleep cycling and arousal. *Pediatr Res,* 1988;24(1):101-105.

18   Mattson SN, Crocker N, Nguyen TT. Fetal Alcohol Spectrum Disorders: Neuropsychological and Behavioral Features. *Neuropsychol Rev.* doi: 10.1007/s11065-011-9167-9, 2011.

19   Jirikowic T, Kartin D, Olson HC. Children with fetal alcohol spectrum disorders: A descriptive profile of adaptive function. *Canadian Journal of Occupational Therapy,* 2008;75(4):238-248.

20   Kodituwakku PW, Kalberg W, May, PA. The effects of prenatal alcohol exposure on executive functioning. *Alcohol Res Health,* 2001;25(3):192-198.

21   Archibald SL, Fennema-Notestine C, Gamst A, Riley EP, Mattson SN, Jernigan, TL. Brain dysmorphology in individuals with severe prenatal alcohol exposure. *Dev Med Child Neurol,* 2001;43(3):148-154.

22 Astley SJ, Aylward EH, Olson HC, Kerns K, Brooks A, Coggins TE, ... Richards, T. Magnetic resonance imaging outcomes from a comprehensive magnetic resonance study of children with fetal alcohol spectrum disorders. *Alcohol Clin Exp Res,* 2009;33(10), 1671-1689. doi: ACER1004 [pii] 10.1111/j.1530-0277.2009.01004.x.

23 Burke MW, Palmour RM, Ervin FR, Ptito M. Neuronal reduction in frontal cortex of primates after prenatal alcohol exposure. *Neuroreport,* 2009;20(1), 13-17. doi: 10.1097/WNR.0b013e32831b449c.

24 Chen X, Coles CD, Lynch ME, Hu X. Understanding specific effects of prenatal alcohol exposure on brain structure in young adults. *Hum Brain Mapp.* doi: 10.1002/hbm.21313, 2011.

25 Clark CM, Li D, Conry J, Conry R, Loock C. Structural and functional brain integrity of fetal alcohol syndrome in nonretarded cases. *Pediatrics,* 2000;105(5), 1096-1099.

26 Coles CD, Lynch ME, Kable JA, Johnson KC, Goldstein FC. Verbal and nonverbal memory in adults prenatally exposed to alcohol. *Alcohol Clin Exp Res,* 2010;34(5), 897-906. doi: ACER1162 [pii] 10.1111/j.1530-0277.2010.01162.x.

27 Cortese BM, Moore GJ, Bailey BA, Jacobson SW, Delaney-Black V, Hannigan JH. Magnetic resonance and spectroscopic imaging in prenatal alcohol-exposed children: preliminary findings in the caudate nucleus. *Neurotoxicol Teratol,* 2006;28(5), 597-606. doi: S0892-0362(06)00087-0 [pii] 10.1016/j.ntt.2006.08.002.

28 Fagerlund A, Heikkinen S, Autti-Ramo I, Korkman M, Timonen M, Kuusi T, ... Lundbom, N. Brain metabolic alterations in adolescents and young adults with fetal alcohol spectrum disorders. *Alcohol Clin Exp Res,* 2006;30(12), 2097-2104. doi: ACER257 [pii] 10.1111/j.1530-0277.2006.00257.x.

29 Fryer SL, Tapert SF, Mattson SN, Paulus MP, Spadoni AD, Riley EP. Prenatal alcohol exposure affects frontal-striatal response during inhibitory control. *Alcohol Clin Exp Res,* 2007;31(8), 1415-1424. doi: ACER443 [pii] 10.1111/j.1530-0277.2007.00443.x.

30 Lebel C, Rasmussen C, Wyper K, Walker L, Andrew G, Yager J, Beaulieu C. Brain diffusion abnormalities in children with fetal alcohol spectrum disorder. *Alcohol Clin Exp Res,* 2008;32(10), 1732-1740. doi: ACER750 [pii] 10.1111/j.1530-0277.2008.00750.x.

31 Mattson SN, Riley EP. Brain anomalies in fetal alcohol syndrome. In E. L. Abel (Ed.), *Fetal alcohol syndrome: From mechanism to prevention* (pp. 51-68). Boca Raton, FL: CRC Press. 1996.

32 Mattson SN, Riley EP, Jernigan TL, Ehlers CL, Delis DC, Jones KL, . . . Bellugi U. Fetal alcohol syndrome: a case report of neuropsychological, MRI and EEG assessment of two children. *Alcohol Clin Exp Res,* 1992;16(5):1001-1003.

33 Nardelli A, Lebel C, Rasmussen C, Andrew G, Beaulieu C. Extensive deep gray matter volume reductions in children and adolescents with fetal alcohol spectrum disorders. *Alcohol Clin Exp Res,* 2011;35(8), 1404-1417. doi: 10.1111/j.1530-0277.2011.01476.x.

34 O'Hare ED, Lu LH, Houston SM, Bookheimer SY, Mattson SN, O'Connor MJ, Sowell ER. Altered frontal-parietal functioning during verbal working memory in children and adolescents with heavy prenatal alcohol exposure. *Hum Brain Mapp,* 2009;30(10):3200-3208. doi: 10.1002/hbm.20741.

35 Roussotte FF, Bramen JE, Nunez SC, Quandt LC, Smith L, O'Connor MJ, . . . Sowell ER. Abnormal brain activation during working memory in children with prenatal exposure to drugs of abuse: the effects of methamphetamine, alcohol, and polydrug exposure. *Neuroimage,* 2011;54(4), 3067-3075. doi: S1053-8119(10)01380-7 [pii].

36 Sowell ER, Leow AD, Bookheimer SY, Smith LM, O'Connor MJ, Kan E, . . . Thompson PM. Differentiating prenatal exposure to methamphetamine and alcohol versus alcohol and not methamphetamine using tensor-based brain morphometry and discriminant analysis. *J Neurosci,* 2010;30(11):3876-3885. doi: 30/11/3876 [pii].

37 Sowell ER, Lu LH, O'Hare ED, McCourt ST, Mattson SN, O'Connor MJ, Bookheimer SY. Functional magnetic resonance imaging of verbal learning in children with heavy prenatal alcohol exposure. *Neuroreport,* 2007;18(7):635-639. doi: 10.1097/WNR.0b013e3280bad8dc 00001756-200705070-00003 [pii].

38 Spadoni AD, Bazinet AD, Fryer SL, Tapert SF, Mattson SN, Riley EP. Response during spatial working memory in youth with heavy prenatal alcohol exposure. *Alcohol Clin Exp Res,* 2009;33(12):2067-2076. doi: ACER1046 [pii] 10.1111/j.1530-0277.2009.01046.x.

39 Willford J, Day R, Aizenstein H, & Day N. Caudate asymmetry: A neurobiological marker of moderate prenatal alcohol exposure in young

adults. *Neurotoxicology and Teratology,* 2010;32(6):589-594. doi: 10.1016/j.ntt.2010.06.012.

40 Haley DW, Handmaker NS, Lowe J. Infant stress reactivity and prenatal alcohol exposure. *Alcohol Clin Exp Res,* 2006;30(12):2055-2064. doi: ACER251 [pii] 10.1111/j.1530-0277.2006.00251.x.

41 Hellemans KG, Sliwowska JH, Verma P, Weinberg JA. Prenatal alcohol exposure: fetal programming and later life vulnerability to stress, depression and anxiety disorders. Neurosci Biobehav Rev, 2010;34(6):791-807. doi: S0149-7634(09)00084-0 [pii]10.1016/j.neubiorev.2009.06.004.

42 Oberlander TF, Jacobson SW, Weinberg JA, Grunau RE, Molteno CD, Jacobson JL. Prenatal alcohol exposure alters biobehavioral reactivity to pain in newborns. *Alcohol Clin Exp Res,* 2010;34(4):681-692. doi: ACER1137 [pii] 10.1111/j.1530-0277.2009.01137.x.

43 Olson HC, Jirikowic T, Kartin D, Astley SJ. Responding to the challenge of early intervention for fetal alcohol spectrum disorders. *Infants & Young Children,* 2007;20(2):172-189.

44 Disney ER, Iacono W, McGue M, Tully E, Legrand L. Strengthening the case: prenatal alcohol exposure is associated with increased risk for conduct disorder. *Pediatrics,* 2008;122(6), e1225-1230. doi: 122/6/e1225 [pii] 10.1542/peds.2008-1380.

45 Nanson JL, Hiscock M. Attention deficits in children exposed to alcohol prenatally. *Alcohol Clin Exp Res,* 1990;14(5):656-661.

46 O'Connor MJ, Paley B. Psychiatric conditions associated with prenatal alcohol exposure. *Dev Disabil Res Rev,* 2009;15(3), 225-234. doi: 10.1002/ddrr.74.

47 Peadon E, Elliott EJ. Distinguishing between attention-deficit hyperactivity and fetal alcohol spectrum disorders in children: clinical guidelines. *Neuropsychiatr Dis Treat,* 2010;6:509-515.

48 Streissguth AP, Bookstein FL, Barr HM, Sampson PD, O'Malley K, & Young JK. Risk factors for adverse life outcomes in fetal alcohol syndrome and fetal alcohol effects. *J Dev Behav Pediatr,* 2004;25(4), 228-238. doi: 00004703-200408000-00002 [pii].

49 Walthall JC, O'Connor MJ, Paley BA. Comparison of psychopathology in children with and without prenatal alcohol exposure. *Mental Health Aspects of Developmental Disabilities,* 2008;11(3):69-78.

50   Baer JS, Ginzler JA, Peterson PL. DSM-IV alcohol and substance abuse and dependence in homeless youth. *J Stud Alcohol,* 2003;64(1):5-14.

51   Barr HM, Bookstein FL, O'Malley KD, Connor PD, Huggins JE, Streissguth AP. Binge Drinking During Pregnancy as a Predictor of Psychiatric Disorders on the Structured Clinical Interview for DSM-IV in Young Adult Offspring. *The American Journal of Psychiatry,* 2006;163(6):1061-1065. doi: 10.1176/appi.ajp.163.6.1061.

52   Yates WR, Cadoret RJ, Troughton EP, Stewart M, Giunta TS. Effect of fetal alcohol exposure on adult symptoms of nicotine, alcohol, and drug dependence. *Alcoholism: Clinical and Experimental Research,* 1998;22(4), 914-920. doi: 10.1097/00000374-199806000-00023.

53   Fast DK, & Conry J. Fetal alcohol spectrum disorders and the criminal justice system. *Dev Disabil Res Rev,* 2009;15(3):250-257. doi: 10.1002/ddrr.66.

54   Streissguth AP, Barr HM, Kogan J, Bookstein FL. Primary and Secondary Disabilities in Fetal Alcohol Syndrome. In A. P. Streissguth & J. Kanter (Eds.), *The Challenge of Fetal Alcohol Syndrome: Overcoming Secondary Disabilities* (pp. 25-39). Seattle, WA: Seattle University of Washington Press., 1997.

55   Kooistra L, Crawford S, Gibbard B, Ramage B, Kaplan BJ. Differentiating attention deficits in children with fetal alcohol spectrum disorder or attention-deficit-hyperactivity disorder. *Dev Med Child Neurol,* 2010;52(2):205-211. doi: DMCN3352 [pii] 10.1111/j.1469-8749.2009.03352.x

56   Coggins TE, Timler GR, Olswang LB. A state of double jeopardy: impact of prenatal alcohol exposure and adverse environments on the social communicative abilities of school-age children with fetal alcohol spectrum disorder. *Lang Speech Hear Serv Sch,* 2007;38(2):117-127. doi: 38/2/117 [pii] 10.1044/0161-1461(2007/012).

57   Thorne JC, Coggins TE, Carmichael Olson H, Astley SJ. Exploring the utility of narrative analysis in diagnostic decision making: picture-bound reference, elaboration, and fetal alcohol spectrum disorders. *J Speech Lang Hear Res,* 2007;50(2):459-474. doi: 50/2/459 [pii] 10.1044/1092-4388(2007/032).

58   Coles CD, Strickland DC, Padgett L, & Bellmoff L. Games that "work": using computer games to teach alcohol-affected children about fire and street safety. *Res Dev Disabil,* 2007;28(5), 518-530. doi: S0891-4222(06)00069-2.

59 Astley SJ. Profile of the first 1,400 patients receiving diagnostic evaluations for fetal alcohol spectrum disorder at the Washington State Fetal Alcohol Syndrome Diagnostic & Prevention Network. *Can J Clin Pharmacol,* 2010;17(1), e132-164.

60 O'Connor MJ, Frankel F, Paley B, Schonfeld AM, Carpenter E, Laugeson EA, Marquardt RA. Controlled social skills training for children with fetal alcohol spectrum disorders. *J Consult Clin Psychol,* 2006;74(4), 639-648. doi: 10.1037/0022-006X.74.4.639.

61 Coles CD, Smith I, Fernhoff PM, Falek A. Neonatal neurobehavioral characteristics as correlates of maternal alcohol use during gestation. *Alcohol Clin Exp Res,* 1985;9(5), 454-460.

62 Aronson M, Lyllerman M, Sabel KG, Sandin B, Olegard R. Children of alcohol mothers. Developmental, perceptual, and behavioural characteristics as compared to matched controls. *Acta Paediatrica Scandinavica,* 1985;74(1):27-35.

63 Janzen LA, Nanson JL, Block GW. Neuropsychological evaluation of preschoolers with fetal alcohol syndrome. *Neurotoxicol Teratol,* 1995;17(3):273-279. doi: 089203629400063J [pii].

64 Kyllerman M, Aronson M, Sabel KG, Karlberg E, Sandin B, Olegard R. Childern of alcohol mothers. Acta Paediatrica Scandinavica, 1985;74:20-26.

65 Barr HM, Streissguth AP, Darby BL, Sampson PD. Prenatal exposure to alcohol, caffeine, tobacco, and aspirin: Effects on fine and gross motor performance n 4-year-old children. *Developmental Psychology,* 1990;26:339-348.

66 Conry J. Neuropsychological deficits in fetal alcohol syndrome and fetal alcohol effects. *Alcohol Clin Exp Res,* 1990;14(5):650-655.

67 Aronson M, Lyllerman M, Sabel KG, Sandin B, & Olegard R. Children of alcohol mothers. Developmental, perceptual, and behavioural characteristics as compared to matched controls. *Acta Paediatrica Scandinavica,* 1985;74(1):27-35.

68 Marcus JC. Neurological findings in the fetal alcohol syndrome. *Neuropediatrics,* 1987;18(3):158-160. doi: 10.1055/s-2008-1052471.

69 Roebuck TM, Simmons RW, Richardson C, Mattson SN, Riley EP. Neuromuscular responses to disturbance of balance in children with

prenatal exposure to alcohol. *Alcohol Clin Exp Res,* 1998;22(9), 1992-1997. doi: 00000374-199812000-00015 [pii].

70   Steinhausen HC, Nestler V, Spohr HL. Development of psychopathology of children with the fetal alcohol syndrome. *J Dev Behav Pediatr,* 1982;3(2):49-54.

71   Conn-Blowers EA. Nurturing and educating children prenatally exposed to alcohol: The role of the counsellor. *International Journal for the Advancement of Counseling,* 1991;14(2):91-103.

72   Lynch ME, Coles CD, Corley T, Falek A. Examining delinquency in adolescents differentially prenatally exposed to alcohol: the role of proximal and distal risk factors. *J Stud Alcohol,* 2003;64(5):678-686.

CHAPTER 3 — *Education*

FASDs, ADOLESCENCE AND SCHOOL

Ron Powell, Ph.D.

Dr. Ron Powell, director of the Desert Mountain SELPA in San Bernardino, California, is a leading advocate for special education services for children and youth with FASDs. In this chapter, he examines the teen in school and the challenges adolescents with prenatal exposure to alcohol often face. He breaks down ways to mitigate some of the cognitive and behavioral deficits found in young people affected by prenatal alcohol exposure and offers educational strategies that parents and teachers can use.

Despite prenatal alcohol exposure's significant role as a public health problem and its implications for school systems, there is a dearth of well-designed intervention studies that can guide the design of effective instructional and educational practices.[1] One possible reason for this lack of attention given to the design of learning strategies for children with FASDs is that there are no standard criteria for the identification of children who manifest the neurodevelopmental effects of prenatal alcohol exposure in the absence of the physical features of fetal alcohol syndrome (FAS).[2] The failure of researchers and policy makers to come to consensus on the core elements of a specific phenotype for children affected by prenatal alcohol exposure results in confusion about both the definition and the diagnostic standards for the identification of children with FASDs. Moreover, while many child advocates argue against the inevitable labeling of the child that would result from clear and specific criteria, unambiguous categorization is essential for research as well as for meeting the service needs of this population. Without clear diagnostic criteria, many children with FASDs "fall through the cracks" in the school system and struggle in the general education setting without being identified for specialized instructional assistance. As a result, the varied nature of the FASDs' pattern of strengths and weaknesses results in a reactive as opposed to a strategic approach to the learning difficulties presented by the child. Service providers and care givers who are uninformed regarding the impact of prenatal alcohol exposure on the central nervous system may view children with FASDs as slow learners, lacking in the motivation or willpower necessary to attend to classroom instruction. This off-the-radar view of the child with FASDs is not unique to schools.

Evidence demonstrates that even in clinical settings that specialize in the provision of services that target developmental and behavioral problems, most children with FASDs are not diagnosed.[3]

INDIVIDUALS WITH DISABILITIES EDUCATION ACT

The Individuals with Disabilities Education Act (IDEA) mandates that school districts actively identify and provide an appropriate education to all children with disabilities who reside within the district's boundaries. Nationally, about 13% of children ages 3 to 21 qualify for special education services.[4] But for children with FASDs, many are found not to qualify under IDEA because their learning problems are not considered to be significant enough to meet the eligibility requirements. For example, children with FASDs commonly experience global delays in cognitive functioning that range in IQ from < 70 for children with FAS to > 85 for children with alcohol related neurodevelopmental disorder (ARND).[5]

Specific eligibility standards, however, for each of the 13 disabilities under IDEA are established by the states. While the definition of intellectual disability under the IDEA includes "significantly subaverage general intellectual functioning," existing concurrently with deficits in adaptive behavior[6] the quantification of "significant subaverage" differs from state to state. In most states, this criterion parallels the definition of mental retardation established by the American Psychiatric Association as a threshold score on a standardized measure of general intellectual functioning (i.e., IQ < 70).[7] Some states, however, follow the more recent guidelines of the American Association on Intellectual and Developmental Disabilities that allow consideration of the standard error of measurement and use IQ < 75[8,9] as the criterion. Similarly, eligibility criteria for Specific Learning Disability as well as Other Health Impaired – the disability category that includes attention deficit disorder (ADD) and attention deficit hyperactivity disorder (ADHD) – vary from state to state. As a result of this variability, many children with FASDs may not qualify for special education services, and of those who do qualify, the specific disability category of an individual student may vary from state to state.

Regardless of whether or not a child with FASDs meets the criteria to qualify for special education services, eligibility as a child with a disability is no guarantee that a child with FASDs will be appropriately served. Special education services under the IDEA include specially designed instruction to meet the unique needs of a child with a disability. Special education services must be specified on an Individualized Education Program (IEP) and must include consideration of related services and necessary supports, modifications and accommodations to provide access to the general education curriculum.[10,11] While special education services generally occur in smaller learning environments that allow for more individualized assistance, without specific training in the unique areas of deficit presented by the child with FASDs, the teacher tends to rely solely on his or her experience in designing instructional interventions rather than on research findings.[1]

A recent observation within a special education classroom illustrates the degree of adaptation that a teacher must be able to make in order to accommodate a child with FASDs.

> *"What do we have to do this stuff for anyway?"*
> *The question had a defiant tone and broke the silence of the classroom. Heads popped up, and then looked down again to the practice worksheets in front of them.*
> *"This stuff is baby!" the voice grew louder. "It's easy! I can do it easy!" The young man slammed his pencil down hard onto the desk and pushed his chair back in now obvious frustration.*
> *"Shut up! I can't think," said the girl to the side, her face still buried in her work.*
> *"You're a baby, Steven," sniped the boy from the back in what was now an escalating disruption.*
> *The teacher began to move toward the young man who was now visibly agitated, counting on proximity control to quiet the disturbance.*

Steven was correct, of course. Simple addition with two columns of numbers was not the type of mathematics problem assigned to his peers. And he also was correct that he had seen this type of problem before. With only one year left in high school, two-column addition had been a part of his math curriculum for many years.

> *As the teacher approached his desk, Steven again yelled, "It's easy! I can do this easy!"*
> *"I know you can," the teacher said in a calm and reassuring tone. The volume of the response was barely above a whisper as the teacher purposefully turned his body to the side and avoided eye contact, using body language to deescalate the situation. "I can see that you don't want to repeat work that you have already done," the teacher said, validating Steven's sense of frustration. "Why don't you grab your book and come meet with me in my office?"*
> *The teacher's response prompted a ripple of laughter across the room and a slight smile from Steven. As a self-contained special education environment, the space was barely large enough for the nine students in the program. The narrow rectangular space was more like a fuselage than a classroom. The "office" was a reference to a chair positioned adjacent to the teacher's desk for individual assistance. The absurdity of the "inside joke" was enough to break the tension and distract Steven for a moment from the rising frustration of the task.*

Like many children with FASDs, Steven faced significant challenges in keeping pace with the rigors of the standard curriculum. Prenatal alcohol exposure is highly correlated with deficits in global cognitive functioning as measured by standard IQ testing.[12] Early studies suggest that some individuals identified with FASDs meet the criteria for intellectual disability, defined in part as an IQ of less than 70.[12,13] Steven met this criterion with a tested IQ of 69. However, Steven's reading level was sufficient to offer him a degree of independence. His grandparents, with whom he had lived since birth, had read to him regularly and his grandfather had established a regular routine of discussing the sports section in the morning paper. Reading at about the fifth grade level allowed Steven to read most of the content in the paper. However, while he could pick out a batting average from the box scores, he had difficulty comprehending the simple computation upon which it was based.

Individuals with cognitive impairment are widely recognized to have difficulties in school and with tasks of everyday living. But children affected by prenatal alcohol exposure experience greater difficulties with memory than can be explained by deficits in global cognitive ability alone. Particularly, they have difficulty with "rote" memory tasks and in encoding new information. They also struggle with employing strategies to facilitate storage into long-term memory. This is especially evident in learning new material or new characteristics of information.[2,14] This characteristic poses a significant problem for learning new information in an academic setting and will require that instructional supports be built into the intervention strategies.

> *Seated next to the teacher and removed from the watchful eyes of his classmates, Steven seemed willing to demonstrate his capacity to solve two-column addition problems. He looked at the first problem (12+14). Steven drew a line across the top of his paper and made hash marks on the line. He then numbered each hash mark from 0 to 10. Using the newly created number line as a tool, Steven marked off the hash marks while saying the numbers aloud. "One, two." He stopped and put his finger on the number "2" as a placeholder. He glanced at the problem again and then began to count off the hash marks using his pencil as a pointer and starting from his finger. "One, Two, Three, Four." He stopped and looked at the number on the number line that was beneath the point of his pencil. "Six" he said confidently, and then wrote a "6" below the line on his problem. He used the same process for adding "1" + "1." As he finished marking the*

"2" on his paper, he looked to the teacher for approval. "What number is that?" asked the teacher. "26" Steven responded, now clearly pleased with himself. "That's correct," affirmed the teacher. "Let's try another one."

What is clear to the teacher is that Steven has learned a strategy for solving an addition problem, but it has limited application. While the strategy may be successful with single column addition when the sum of the numbers is less than "10," it is not going to be a successful strategy for solving problems that require regrouping. Steven, however, has learned a strategy to the point of mastery and is able to retrieve that strategy whenever he is presented with an addition problem. This now poses a dilemma for the teacher. Should the teacher try to adapt the "number line" strategy that Steven has already learned in order to make it appropriate for more difficult problems, or should the teacher try to engage Steven in a new strategy that is more effective?

Research on memory with the FASDs population provides insight into the teacher's observations of Steven's learning difficulties. Children who have been affected by prenatal exposure to alcohol process information more slowly than typical individuals[15-19] because of the adverse effect of alcohol on the hippocampus, the frontal lobe, and the white matter integrity of the brain.[14,20,21] The slower flow of information processing makes it more difficult for the child with FASDs to hold and process information in working memory.[22,23] In addition, children with FASDs experience significant difficulty with visual-spatial memory[23] and have been shown to have particular difficulty with basic numerical processing which includes the ability to mentally represent and manipulate numbers and quantities.[24] Steven's strategy of holding his finger or the point of his pencil on the number line was a compensatory strategy to accommodate for this deficit. Although Steven struggled with remembering the sum of his computation long enough to write the answer on his paper, the strategy of the number line had been learned to mastery, and he was able to easily retrieve the strategy to apply to the problem. Studies support this observation, noting that for children with

FASDs, once information has been learned to mastery, it is retained as effectively as in typical peers.[25] Thus, the primary difficulty with learning new material seems to be with input of information rather than with retrieval.

The unique quality of this memory deficit is readily demonstrated with a simple example. Imagine, if you were asked to repeat a string of six random numbers like "716942". Most people would be able to hear the string of numbers and immediately reproduce the list with accuracy. But, imagine how much more difficult this task would be if the presentation of the stimulus was modified by spacing each number in the sequence two minutes apart from the next. Since the twelve-minute span between the presentation of the first number and the appointed time for the recital of the list exceeds the working memory of most individuals, you would probably need to employ some type of memory strategy to aid in the retention of the sequence. Perhaps you would mentally rehearse the numbers repeatedly or combine the numbers into clusters of two or three digits, or connect the numbers to dates with which you are already familiar. Now imagine if you were trying to complete this task while talking on the telephone or texting. The presence of distractions that require thought further compromises the capacity of the brain to work with information that has yet to be stored into long-term memory.

DEFICITS IN ATTENTION

This example captures the experience of the child with FASDs in trying to make meaning of new information. A constant barrage of stimuli from the environment overwhelms the slower processing speed of the brain. Moreover, when inefficient learning strategies are coupled with deficits in attention, the inability to filter out extraneous sensory input through concentration on only salient information further complicates the young person's efforts to learn. This is a common problem for children with FASDs although the mechanism of the attention problem is not fully understood.[26]

Attention deficit disorder (ADD) and attention deficit hyperactivity disorder (ADHD) are diagnosed in more than 70% of all alcohol-exposed children.[27,28] But some researchers believe that the reason that children with

FASDs have difficulty sustaining attention and maintaining concentration relates more heavily to deficits in arousal and self-regulation rather than with impulse control.[28-31] It is not surprising then, that evidence points to a connection between arousal regulation in children with FASDs and deficits in self-control and behavioral regulation. If alcohol-exposed children are more easily aroused to environmental stimuli, but have difficulty moderating the state of arousal once it is activated, then sustaining attention on a task becomes more difficult and learning cannot occur efficiently.[18,19]

EXECUTIVE FUNCTIONING

Deficits in short term memory, attention, and arousal regulation combine to further compromise the processing of information through higher-order cognitive processes. The frontal lobe of the brain is the center for executive functioning. Executive functioning includes the regulation of attention and the processing of information through working memory as well as planning, organization, and problem-solving.[32] Most sensory information travels from the respective receptive centers in the brain to the frontal lobe for processing. Since we would easily be overwhelmed if our brain retained every bit of information that our senses pick up, the brain must make a determination of which information is important to bring to our attention or to retain, and which information to ignore. Our ability to learn from experience, to plan for an event or to be on time to a business meeting or family dinner are all dependent on executive functioning.[33,34]

Working memory plays an especially important part in the efficiency and effectiveness of executive functioning. Working memory allows us to hold units of information in short term memory simultaneously so that they can be evaluated, ordered, synthesized, discarded, or reorganized to enable the best decisions among alternatives to be determined.[35]

The negative impact that prenatal alcohol exposure has on executive functioning and particularly working memory accounts for much of the cognitive impairment evident in this population.[22] Children with FASDs have been shown to perform more poorly than controls on planning tasks and to repeatedly respond incorrectly, thus demonstrating difficulty in learning from mistakes and adapting responses based upon environmental cues.[20,22,36] This resistance to new patterns and strategies in preference for inefficient learned responses complicates the role of the teacher in the presentation of new techniques for processing information. It also emphasizes the high stakes involved in choosing teaching strategies that accommodate the unique pattern of strengths and weaknesses that characterize the learning behavior of children with FASDs.

FAMILY-BASED INTERVENTIONS

Little systematic research has been devoted to understanding effective behavioral interventions[1] or educational strategies for children with FASDs.[37] Although an extensive body of research exists regarding the etiology and manifestations of the impact of prenatal alcohol exposure,[38,39] few empirically supported interventions can be found.[40,41] Empirically supported interventions are those that meet scientific standards for rigor and design that are judged sufficient to determine unequivocally that the effects of treatment are not the result of chance or other confounding factors.[42-44] A comprehensive search of the research literature identified only 12 published intervention studies for children with FASDs that met this standard of scientific rigor.[45-47] These intervention studies focused on the treatment of diverse deficits within the areas of cognitive and adaptive behavior skills.[41] A review of these studies reveals mixed results, with some studies showing minimal treatment gains and others hampered by small sample size.[41,48] However, an important conclusion that can be drawn from this limited set of studies is that interventions can be effective in ameliorating some of the behavioral and learning deficits caused by prenatal alcohol exposure. In reviewing five of these studies, Bertrand and colleagues[49] identified two factors that emerge as important contributors to effective outcomes: the inclusion of a parent training component and the direct instruction of skills.

Families are a vital part of the success of any treatment effort. Children with FASDs who are raised from an early age in stable and loving homes experience more positive life outcomes than children who are not raised in such supportive environments.[50] Similarly, children with FASDs who did not report disrupted school experiences (i.e., suspensions, expulsions, or drop out) attributed their positive experience to the fact that they had made a connection with someone at school who really cared about them.[51] Correspondingly, similar findings exist within the educational literature as it relates to the effects of the teacher-student relationship on academic performance. Cornelius-White[52] examined the impact of the relationship between the teacher and the student and found that 76% of students who reported positive relationships with their teachers demonstrated significantly more positive academic outcomes as well as improved attitudes in school compared to students who did not report positive relationships with their teachers. For this reason, school and community resources need to be provided that assist the family in reducing stress and increasing positive interactions within the home through the provision of physical and psychological resources.[53] Three of the evidence-based interventions reviewed by Bertrand employed a family training component that may hold promise for the reduction of problem behaviors: Neurocognitive Habilitation,[54] Parent Child Interaction Therapy (PCIT), and a behavioral consultation program called Families Moving Forward (FMF).[49]

The Neurocognitive Habilitation program utilized a group treatment approach to improve the executive functioning and emotional regulation of the child with FASDs. The program assisted the child to recognize and monitor his arousal and activity level by using the metaphor of a car engine. The activities were structured to build upon the child's strengths, and new skills were consistently reinforced and expanded with opportunities to rehearse and generalize skills within multiple contexts. The curriculum was implemented in 75-minute sessions over a 12-week period. Parent education sessions were held concurrently with the treatment sessions in which the parents received training on how to recognize and respond to the emotional and behavioral changes that their child demonstrated. Parents were taught to utilize strategies that were appropriate for the child's developmental level and that engaged the child in meaningful interactive activities. Children who participated in the program made significant improvements in executive and emotional functioning compared to the control group.[54]

Parent Child Interaction Therapy (PCIT)[49] is a dyadic therapeutic approach that draws upon operant conditioning and play therapy to address challenging behaviors.[55,56] PCIT allows parents to interact directly with their child in treatment while the parents are provided in-vivo coaching through an in-ear communication device from a therapist observing the session from another room. Treatment consists of parenting skills (i.e., reinforcement and praise skills, setting of boundaries, active ignoring, etc.) as well as reinforcement and support of parental progress as they become more proficient in utilizing the skills. PCIT sessions were held weekly over a 14-week period. The PCIT treatment group was compared to a control group that received parenting support in the form of education about child development as well as training about general behavior management techniques. The results of the study showed that children in both the treatment as well as the control group demonstrated a significant decrease in challenging behaviors as well as a decrease in parental stress among the caregivers.

The goal of the Families Moving Forward program (FMF)[49] was to reduce the challenging behavior of the child with FASDs by providing parent training in strategies that work with children with FASDs as well as supportive behavioral consultation. Training was provided in 90-minute sessions held every-other-week over a 9 to 11 month period. Upon completion of the treatment, the FMF group demonstrated a significant reduction of challenging behaviors as well as an increased sense of parental self-efficacy compared to the control group. There was no difference, however, between the two groups in regard to parental stress level.

While these three studies were divergent in the degree to which they provided direct intervention with the child, they all proved to be successful in the extent to which problem behaviors were reduced and parents expressed satisfaction with the program. Involvement of parents in the treatment of the child has been broadly recognized as an important tool in addressing the behavior challenges of the child.[57-59] Given that the behavior of the child with FASDs is pervasive across multiple environments, and that reduction in stress within the environment is important to foster self regulatory control, it is vital that the caregivers be provided with training and resources that will allow them to act as partners in the process of supporting the child's efforts to develop appropriate regulatory controls.

SCHOOL-BASED INTERVENTION STRATEGIES

The description of the unique profile of cognitive skills observed among children with prenatal alcohol exposure has begun to crystallize around a consensus view that cognitive performance among children with FASDs is characterized by a generalized deficit in the processing and integration of multiple elements or relationships among units of information.[60-63] As a result, information is processed slowly, and particular difficulty is evident with performance on complex tasks that involve executive control.[60,61] This conceptualization has been found to differentiate children prenatally exposed to alcohol from non-exposed controls across all FASDs subtypes including higher functioning children without intellectual disability.[64]

It remains to be seen whether conceptualizing FASDs in this way simplifies and broadens the diagnostic protocol for the identification of FASDs. But understanding the cognitive and behavioral characteristics of FASDs from the perspective that they are manifestations of central nervous system damage that impair the ability of the child to process and integrate information may be helpful within the educational environment in the early identification and design of educational and therapeutic interventions that address these deficits. Streissguth et. al.[50] report that early identification is a vital protective factor against the adverse life outcomes common to children with FASDs, including trouble with the law, alcohol and drug problems, and imprisonment. These problems have been shown to increase with age and persist into adulthood. This life course trajectory originates during the time children with FASDs are in school and affects males in a much more dramatic way than females. Males are more likely than females to have difficulty in school (67%) and to experience trouble with the law and confinement. Moreover, the lack of resources to assist children in schools is positively linked to both incarceration as well as trouble with the law. Of those males with difficulty in school, 83% also reported trouble with the law and 69% of these males were incarcerated.[50] In contrast, increased availability of support services to assist children affected by prenatal alcohol exposure to be successful in school is negatively correlated with trouble with the law. Similarly, early diagnosis and the provision of support services in schools together with the enduring presence of a stable and nurturing home environment were negatively correlated to the occurrence and severity of alcohol/drug problems in adolescence and adulthood.[50] The challenge for schools, then, is to structure an environment that scaffolds supports within the classroom to accommodate the slower processing speed and information processing deficits of the child with FASDs.

Given the paucity of intervention studies that address the educational experience for adolescents with FASDs, in order to design structures and supports that ensure that adolescents with FASDs succeed in their school experience we are left to connect our knowledge of their processing deficits with strategies that have been shown to work with individuals with similar deficits. Certainly, the presentation of information in smaller increments and at a slower pace makes sense in order to accommodate the working memory deficits of the child with FASDs. Furthermore, using concrete examples, manipulatives, and project-based learning have been found to be successful strategies for individuals who have difficulty with abstract concepts and generalization to "real world" experience. But the key for academic content is the presentation of material in a way that accommodates the memory deficits of the student.

DIRECT INSTRUCTION

One of the most powerful learning strategies for both general education students as well as students with disabilities is Direct Instruction.[65] Direct Instruction has seven major steps:

1. Clearly identify what the learning intentions are, i.e., what the child will be able to do as a result of the instruction.
2. Identify the success criteria and inform the student about the standards of performance.
3. Build commitment and engagement by using a "hook" to focus attention and draw the student into the lesson.

4. Present the lesson using small increments of information that build upon prior knowledge and scaffold to higher understanding. Model how to practice the skill. Re-teach if necessary to ensure that the student is practicing the skill or concept correctly.
5. Provide for guided practice under the supervision of the teacher who moves around the room checking for understanding.
6. Bring the lesson to closure by reviewing and clarifying key points to the lesson. The skill or concept is integrated into the whole to ensure that the student has integrated the concept into a larger conceptual network.
7. Provide the opportunity for independent practice. This step allows the student to practice the skill that has been mastered for the purpose of reinforcement and over-learning. This step is used to generalize the concept to a variety of other contexts, employing a range of reinforcement practice opportunities.

Direct Instruction has been found to be effective for general education students[50] as well as special education students[66-68] and has many of the elements that are important for accommodating the learning deficits of children with FASDs. By providing explicit instruction in the concept or skill to be taught and offering guided supports to ensure that the child has mastered the subject before given time to practice independently, the structure of the lesson presentation assists the child in maintaining attention without becoming frustrated with the task.

MNEMONIC INSTRUCTION

Another powerful instructional strategy is mnemonic instruction.[69] Mnemonic instruction aids in the acquisition of information by teaching the child to utilize visual or verbal pegs to facilitate the encoding as well as recall of information. The methodology has proven to be successful with students with disabilities to assist in the memorization of lists that are common tasks in content classes at the secondary level. For example, mnemonic strategies have been shown to assist with the recall of states and their capitals and the list of minerals and their common characteristics on the hardness scale. Mnemonics in the form of acrostics are also common for memorizing lists (e.g. HOMES: the great lakes Huron, Ontario, Michigan, Erie and Superior or "Please excuse my dear Aunt Sally" (the order of operations in mathematics).

The learning difficulties of children and adolescents with FASDs are complex.[70] Affected youth often experience problems with social interaction and peer relationships, but given proper supports in school, they generally do not experience debilitating conduct problems[70,71] They exhibit processing deficits[72,73] and significant difficulties in math,[74-76] but have been assessed with cognitive abilities that generally fall within the normal range.[77] And while nearly 70% of youth with FASDs are identified with attention problems, only 40% reported having received special education services at some point in their school experience while 65% received remedial help.[77] It is not uncommon, given the diverse range of academic and behavioral deficits, that the needs of children with FASDs frequently are not taken seriously in the schools. School personnel may misinterpret the learning difficulties as a lack of motivation or a matter of will and not provide the empathy or additional help that the child requires.[78] In some cases, however, the student has come to depend on individualized help, refusing to try for fear of failure. In other cases, like Steven, the student may hide behind bravado in the hope that lack of competence in a skill will not be discovered. While teachers recognize the student as struggling, they lack the knowledge for how to modify their instruction to accommodate the child given the level of responsibility that they have for other students in the classroom.[3] But these challenges do not have to be borne by school personnel alone. As we have seen, involving the parents as partners in the process doubles the efforts of the schools to engage the child in a comprehensive system that works together to meet the needs of the child. If there is a common theme in the complex task of educating the child with FASDs, it lies in the power of collaboration among all those who are involved in the child's life. Doing so will ensure that with sufficient structure and accommodations, adolescents with FASDs are able to graduate from high school and lead satisfying and fulfilling lives.[79-81]

NOTES

1   Kodituwakku PW. A neurodevelopmental framework for the development of interventions for children with fetal alcohol spectrum disorders. *Alcohol.* 2010;44:717-728.

2   Coles CD. Discriminating the effects of prenatal alcohol exposure from other behavioral and learning disorders. *Alcohol Research and Health.* 2011;34:42-50.

3   Ryan A, Ferguson D. On, yet under the radar: Students with fetal alcohol syndrome disorder. *Exceptional Children.* 2006;72:363-379.

4   U.S. Department of Education, National Center for Education Statistics. *Digest of Education Statistics.* 2012 (NCES 2014-015), Chapter 2, (2013).

5   Streissguth AP, Randels SP, Smith DF. A test-retest study of intelligence in patients with fetal alcohol syndrome: Implications for care. *Journal of the American Academy of Child and Adolescent Psychiatry.* 1991;30:584-587.

6   Child With a Disability, 34 C.F.R. Sect.300.8 (c) (6), 2004.

7   *Diagnostic and Statistical Manual of Mental Disorders, Fourth Edition, Text Revision.* 2000; Washington DC, American Psychiatric Association.

8   Grossman H. *Classification in Mental Retardation.* 1983. Washington DC: American Association on Mental Deficiency.

9   Luckasson R, Borthwick-Duffy S, Buntinx WHE, Coulter DL, Craig EM, Reeve A, Shalock RL, Snell ME, Spitalnik DM, Spreat S, Tassé MJ. 2002. *Mental retardation: Definition, classification, and systems of supports.* 10th ed. Washington (DC): American Association on Mental Retardation.

10   Individuals with Disabilities Education Act (IDEA), 34 CFR §300.34 (a). 2004.

11   Individuals with Disabilities Education Act (IDEA), 34 CFR §300.39 (b) (3). 2004.

12   Committee on Substance Abuse and Committee on Children with Disabilities. Fetal alcohol syndrome and alcohol-related neurodevelopmental disorders. *Pediatrics.* 2000;106:358-361.

13 Institute of Medicine (US). Division of Biobehavioral Sciences and Mental Disorders. Committee to Study Fetal Alcohol Syndrome. Stratton K, Howe C, Battaglia F. *Fetal Alcohol Syndrome: Diagnosis, Epidemiology, Prevention and Treatment*. Washington DC: National Academic Press, 1996.

14 Coles CD, Lynch ME, Kable JA, Johnson KC, Goldstein FC. Verbal and nonverbal memory in adults prenatally exposed to alcohol. *Alcoholism: Clinical and Experimental Research*. 2010;34(5):897-906.

15 Jacobson SW, Jacobson JL, Sokol RJ, Martier SS, Ager JW. Prenatal alcohol exposure and infant information processing ability. *Child Development*. 1993;64:1706-1721.

16 Jacobson SW, Jacobson JL, Sokol RJ. Effects of fetal alcohol exposure on infant reaction time. *Alcoholism: Clinical and Experimental Research*. 1994;18:1125-1132.

17 Li L, Coles CD, Lynch ML, Hu X. Voxelwise and skeleton-based region of interest analysis of fetal alcohol syndrome disorders in young adults. *Human Brain Mapping*. 2009;30:3265-3274

18 Coles CD, Platzman KA, Lynch ME, Freides D. Auditory and visual sustained attention in adolescents prenatally exposed to alcohol. *Alcoholism: Clinical and Experimental Research*. 2002;26:263-271.

19 Connor PD, Streissguth AP, Sampson PD. Individual differences in auditory and visual attention among fetal alcohol-affected adults. *Alcoholism: Clinical and Experimental Research*. 1999;23:1395-1402.

20 Kerns KA, Don A, Mateer CA, Streissguth AP. Cognitive deficits in nonretarded adults with fetal alcohol syndrome. *Journal of Learning Disabilities*. 1997;30:685-693.

21 Roebuck-Spencer TM, Mattson SN. Implicit strategy effects learning in children with heavy prenatal alcohol exposure. *Alcoholism: Clinical and Experimental Research*. 2004;28:1424-1431.

22 Kodituwakku PW, Handmaker NS, Cutler SK, Weathersby EK, Handmaker SD. Specific impairments in self-regulation in children exposed to alcohol prenatally. *Alcoholism: Clinical and Experimental Research*. 1995;19:1558-1564.

23 Green CR, Mihic AM, Nikkel SM, Stade BC, Rasmussen C, Munoz DP, et al. Executive function deficits in children with fetal alcohol spectrum

disorders (FASDs) measured using the Cambridge Neuropsychological Tests Automated battery (CANTAB). *Journal of Child Psychology and Psychiatry.* 2009;50(6):688-697.

24 Jacobson JL, Dodge NC, Burden MJ, Klorman R, Jacobson SW. Number processing in adolescents with prenatal alcohol exposure and ADHD: Differences in the neurobehavioral phenotype. *Alcoholism: Clinical and Experimental Research.* 2011;35(3):431-442.

25 Mattson SN, Roebuck TM. Acquisition and retention of verbal and nonverbal information in children with heavy prenatal alcohol exposure. *Alcoholism: Clinical and Experimental Research.* 2002;26:875-882.

26 O'Malley KD, Nanson J. Clinical implications of a link between fetal alcohol spectrum disorder and attention-deficit hyperactivity disorder. *Canadian Journal of Psychiatry.* 2002;47: 349-354.

27 Dalen K, Bruaroy S, Wentzel-Larsen T, Laegreid LM. Cognitive functioning in children prenatally exposed to alcohol and psychotropic drugs. *Neuropediatrics.* 2009; 40:162-167.

28 Burd L, Klug MG, Martsolf JT, Kerbeshian J. Fetal alcohol syndrome: Neuropsychiatric phenomics. *Neurotoxicology and Teratology.* 2003;25:687-705.

29 Nanson JL, Hisock M. Attention deficits in children exposed to alcohol prenatally. *Alcoholism: Clinical and Experimental Research.* 1990;14:656-661.

30 Osterheld JR, Wilson A. ADHD and FAS (Letter to the editor). *Journal of the American Academy of Child and Adolescent Psychiatry.* 1997;36:1163.

31 Kable JA, Coles CD. The impact of prenatal alcohol exposure on neurophysiological encoding of environmental events at six months. *Alcoholism: Clinical and Experimental Research.* 2004;28:489-496.

32 Morris RD. Relationships and distinctions among the concepts of attention, memory and executive function: A developmental perspective. In Lyon GR, Krasnegor N, Eds. *Attention, Memory, and Executive Function.* Baltimore, MD: Paul Brookes Publishing. 1996:11-16.

33 Welsh MC, Pennington BF. Assessing frontal lobe functioning in children: Views from developmental psychology. *Developmental Neuropsychology.* 1988;4(3):199-230.

34   Pennington BF, Ozonoff S. Executive functions and developmental psychopathology. *Journal of Child Psychology and Psychiatry and Allied Disciplines.* 1996;37(1):51-87.

35   Burden MJ, Jacobson SW, Sokol RJ, Jacobson JL. Effects of prenatal alcohol exposure on attention and working memory at 7.5 years of age. *Alcoholism: Clinical and Experimental Research.* 2005;29(3):443-452.

36   Coles CD, Platzman KA, Raskind-Hood CL, Brown RT, Falek A, Smith IE. A comparison of children affected by prenatal alcohol exposure and attention deficit, hyperactivity disorder. *Alcoholism: Clinical and Experimental Research.* 1997;21:150-161.

37   Streissguth AP, Aase JM, Clarren SK, Randels SP, LaDue RA, Smith DF. Fetal alcohol syndrome in adolescents and adults. *JAMA.* 1991;265: 1961-1967.

38   Lemoine P, Harousseau H, Borteyru JP, Menuet JC. Les enfants des parents alcoholiques: anomailes observees a propos de 127 cas. *Quest Medical.* 1968;25:476-487.

39   Jones KL, Smith DW. Recognition of the fetal alcohol syndrome in early infancy. *Lancet.* 1973;2(7836): 999-1001.

40   Kalberg WO, Buckley D. FASDs: What types of intervention and rehabilitation are useful? *Neuroscience and Biobehavioral Reviews.* 2007;31:278-285.

41   Paley B, O'Connor MJ. Interventions for individuals with fetal alcohol spectrum disorders: Treatment approaches and case management. *Developmental Disabilities Research Reviews.* 2009;15(3):258-267.

42   Kazdin, AE. *Research Design in Clinical Psychology* (4th ed). 2002; Boston: Allyn & Bacon

43   Campbell DT, Stanley JC. *Experimental and Quasi-experimental Designs for Research.* Chicago:Rand McNally, 1963.

44   Chambliss DL, Hollon SD. Defining empirically supported therapies. *Journal of Consulting and Clinical Psychology.* 1998;66(1):7-18.

45   Premji S, Benzies K, Serrett K, Hayden KA. Research-based interventions for children and youth with a fetal alcohol spectrum disorder: Revealing the gap. *Child: Care, Health and Development.* 2007;33(4): 389-397. discussion 398-400.

46   Peadon E, Rhys-Jones B, Bower C, Elliott EJ. Systematic review of interventions for children with fetal alcohol spectrum disorders. *BMC Pediatrics.* 2009;9:35.

47   Kodituwakku PW, Kodituwakku EL. From research to practice: An integrative framework for the development of interventions for children with fetal alcohol spectrum disorders. *Neuropsychology Review.* 2011;21(2):204-23.

48   Kodituwakku PW, Kodituwakku EL. From research to practice: An integrative framework for the development of interventions for children with fetal alcohol spectrum disorders. *Neuropsychology Review.* 2011;21(2):204-23.

49   Bertrand J. Interventions for children with fetal alcohol spectrum disorders (FASDs): Overview of findings for five innovative research projects. *Research in Developmental Disabilities.* 2009;30(5):986-1006.

50   Streissguth AP, Bookstein FL, Barr HM, Sampson PD, O'Malley KO, Young JK. Risk factors for adverse life outcomes in fetal alcohol syndrome and fetal alcohol effects. *Developmental and Behavioral Pediatrics.* 2004;25:228-238.

51   Streissguth AP, *Fetal Alcohol Syndrome: A Guide for Families and Communities.* Baltimore MD: Paul H. Brookes, 1997.

52   Cornelius-White, J., Learner-centered teacher-student relationships are effective: A meta-analysis. *Review of Educational Research,* 2007;77(1), 113-143.

53   Guralnick MJ. Effectiveness of early intervention for vulnerable children: A developmental perspective. *American Journal of Mental Retardation.* 1998;102(4):319-345.

54   Wells AM, Chasnoff IJ, Schmidt CA, Telford E, Schwartz LD. Neurocognitive habilitation therapy for children with fetal alcohol spectrum disorders: An adaptation of the Alert Program®. *American Journal of Occupational Therapy.* 2012;66:24-34.

55   Eyberg SM, Matarazzo RG. Training parents as therapists: A comparison between individual parent-child interaction training and parent group didactic training. *Journal of Clinical Psychology.* 1980;36(2):492-499.

56   Eyberg SM, Boggs SR. Parent-child interaction therapy for oppositional preschoolers. In Shaefer CE, Briesmeister JM, (eds). *Handbook of Parent Training: Parents as Co-Therapists Children's Behavior Problems* (2nd ed., pp 61-97), New York, Wiley, 1998.

57   Patterson GR, McNeal N, Hawkins N, Phelps R. Reprogramming the social environment. *Journal of Child Psychology and Psychiatry.* 1967;8:181-195.

58   Schrepfeman L, Snyder J. Coercion: The link between treatment mechanisms in behavioral parent training and risk reduction in child antisocial behavior. *Behavior Therapy.* 2002;33:339-359.

59   Price JM, Chamberlain P, Landsverk J, Reid JB, Leve LD, Laurent H. Effects of a foster parent training intervention on placement changes of children in foster care. *Child Maltreatment.* 2008;13:64-75

60   Kodituwakku PW. Defining the behavioral phenotype in children with fetal alcohol spectrum disorders: A review. *Neuroscience and Biobehavioral Reviews.* 2007;31:192-201.

61   Kodituwakku PW. Neurocognitive profile in children with fetal alcohol spectrum disorders. *Developmental Disability Research Reviews.* 2009;15:218-224.

62   Kodituwakku PW. Is there a behavioral phenotype in children with fetal alcohol spectrum disorders? Shapiro BK, Accardo PJ (eds.). *Neurogenetic Syndromes:Behavioral Issues and their Treatment.* Baltimore MD: Brookes Publishing Co., 2010.

63   Kodituwakku PW, Segall JM, Beatty GK. Cognitive and behavioral effects of prenatal alcohol exposure. *Future Neurology.* 2011;6(2):237-259.

64   Quattlebaum JL, O'Connor MJ. Higher functioning children with prenatal alcohol exposure: Is there a specific neurocognitive profile? *Child Neuropsychology.* 2013;19(6):561-578.

65   Adams GL, Englemann S. *Research on direct instruction: 20 years beyond DISTAR.* Seattle WA: Educational Achievement Systems, 1996.

66   Forness SR, Kavale KA, Blum IM, Lloyd JW. Mega-analysis of meta-analysis. *Teaching Exceptional Children.* 1997;29(6):4-9.

67   Forness SR, Kavale KA. *Efficacy of special education and related services.* Washington D.C.: American Association on Mental Retardation, 1999.

68   Lloyd JW, Forness SR, Kavale KA. Some methods are more effective than others. *Intervention in School and Clinic.* 1998;33:195-200.

69   Mastropieri M, Scruggs T. Constructing more meaningful relationships: Mnemonic instruction for special populations. *Educational Psychology Review.* 1989;1(2);83-111.

70   Howell KK, Lynch ME, Platzman KA, Smith GH, Coles CD. Prenatal alcohol exposure and ability, academic achievement, and school functioning in adolescence: A longitudinal follow-up. *Journal of Pediatric Psychology.* 2005;31(1):116-126.

71   Streissguth AP, Kanter J. *The challenge of fetal alcohol syndrome: Overcoming secondary disabilities.* Seattle: University of Washington Press, 1997.

72   Kerns J, Don A, Mateer C, Streissguth AP. Cognitive deficits in nonretarded adults with fetal alcohol syndrome. *Journal of Learning Disabilities.* 1997;30:685-693.

73   Jacobson SW, Specificity of neurobehavioral outcomes associated with prenatal alcohol exposure. *Alcoholism, Clinical and Experimental Research.* 1998;22: 313-320.

74   Kopera-Frye K, Dehaene S, Streissguth AP. Impairments of number processing induced by prenatal alcohol exposure. *Neuropsychologia.* 1996;34:1187-1196.

75   Meintjes EM, Jacobson JL, Molteno CD, Gatenby JC, Warton C, Cannistraci CJ, et al. An FMRI study of number processing in children with fetal alcohol syndrome. *Alcoholism, Clinical and Experimental Research.* 2010;34(8): 1450-1464.

76   Kable JA, Coles CD, Taddeo E. Sociocognitive habilitation using the Math Interactive Learning Experience (MILE) program for alcohol affected children. *Alcoholism: Clinical and Experimental Research.* 2004;28:489-496.

77   Streissguth AP, Barr H, Kogan J, Bookstein F. *Understanding the occurrence of secondary disabilities in clients with fetal alcohol syndrome (FAS) and fetal alcohol effects (FAE): Final report to the centers for disease control and prevention on Grant No. R04/CCR008515* (Tech. Report No 96060). Seattle: University of Washington Fetal Alcohol and Drug Unit, 1996.

78   Pei J, Job JM, Poth C, Atkinson E. Assessment for intervention of children with fetal alcohol spectrum disorders: Perspectives of classroom

teachers, administrators, caregivers, and allied professionals. *Psychology.* 2012;4(3A): 325-334.

79 Duquette C, Stodel E, Fullarton S, Hagglund K. Persistence in high school: Experiences of adolescents and yound adults with fetal alcohol spectrum disorder. *Journal of Intellectual and Developmental Disability.* 2006;31:219-231.

80 Duquette C, Stodel E, Fullarton S, Hagglund K. Teaching students with developmental disabilities: Tips from teens and young adults with fetal alcohol spectrum disorder. *Teaching Exceptional Children.* 39;28-31.

81 Green JH. Fetal alcohol spectrum disorder: Understanding the effects of prenatal alcohol exposure and supporting students. *Journal of School Health.* 2007;77:103-108.

CHAPTER 4 — *Therapy*

THE PERFECT STORM: COMPLEXITY OF SEXUAL BEHAVIORS IN ADOLESCENTS WITH FASDs

Jenae Holtz, L.M.F.T.

In this chapter, Jenae Holtz, the Director of The Desert Mountain Children's Center in Apple Valley, California, provides an overview of sexuality in adolescents with FASDs and explores the root causes as to why they often act out sexually. Ms. Holtz offers guidance to parents regarding what they should know about educating and protecting youth affected by prenatal alcohol exposure.

Kristin's parents, Bill and Sue, first brought her to Desert Mountain Counseling Center when she was five years old. She was petite and shy with a guarded smile. Kristin had recently been adopted, and although her parents were thrilled to enhance their family with this little one, they also were concerned with some of her behavior and the difficulty she seemed to be having with "attaching" emotionally and physically to them.

The parents were informed by the social worker that Kristin had been prenatally exposed to alcohol. After Kristin's birth, she was neglected, malnourished, and physically and sexually abused by her biological mother and her boyfriend. At the age of four, Kristin was removed from her home and placed in foster care. After several months in foster care, Bill and Sue finally adopted her. Kristin's new parents described her as easily distracted and frequently irritable. Although Kristin had made a few friends with girls in her kindergarten class, she was often awkward with other children and seen as "different." She seemed more comfortable with adults but at the same time, Bill and Sue did not feel that she was able to connect with them as most five-year-olds would.

In addition to what Bill and Sue shared about Kristin's early life events, a complete assessment of Kristin indicated she was struggling with bonding resulting from an early history of trauma, neglect, and abuse. In addition, Kristin was having difficulty in regulating her emotions and was having several sensory issues such as being a very picky eater due to the textures of food and difficulty wearing clothes of certain fabrics with tags. The medical examination confirmed Kristin had the growth and facial anomalies associated with Fetal Alcohol Syndrome (FAS). As a result of the assessments, the main areas of treatment recommended by the comprehensive transdisciplinary team were mental health services in the form of attachment therapy and occupational therapy to address the sensory concerns. The family completed therapy, with the parents learning how to respond differently to Kristin by using description in their communication and by changing their communication style from asking questions to relating to the activity and having conversation around the activity. The key to the therapy was to provide the parents with the tools to positively interact with their child. After two years, Kristin and her parents met their treatment goals.

Several years later, Bill and Sue contacted the agency regarding Kristin's sexual "acting out" behaviors. At the age of ten, Kristin had begun to find ways to communicate with older men through the computer, cell phone, and social engagements. She began to sneak out of the house, meeting "friends" in various places (often at the older man's house). Kristin began to engage in sexual relationships with men over the age of 18 years old. By the time Kristin returned to treatment at age twelve, she had run away from home several times and was active sexually with several men whom she professed to "love."

Kristin's parents were beyond worried with their daughter's behaviors. They had taken extreme measures to protect their daughter by installing a security system in the home, taking turns with remaining awake to ensure their daughter would not leave the home, and removing Kristin's access to the computer and cell phone. Nevertheless, Kristin continued to find ways to contact men through peers at church and at school. She continued to be impulsive and make poor decisions. When questioned about her choices, Kristin was able to acknowledge inappropriate behaviors and feel remorse for decisions she was making although her behavior was not changing.

SEXUAL BEHAVIORS IN TEENS WITH FASDs
All teens, including those with Fetal Alcohol Spectrum Disorders, are inundated with hormones, mood changes and overall chaos within their social and emotional lives. The link between FASDs and age-related impairments has prompted increased attention to the associated developmental disabilities that are characterized by physical, cognitive and behavioral impairments.[1] Many children and adolescents diagnosed with FASDs exhibit behaviors such as irritability, lying, stealing, aggressive behaviors, impulsiveness, poor academics, poor decision making and inappropriate sexual behaviors (though, these behaviors may apply to typical teens as well). Adolescents with FASDs show typical indicators of being "risk takers" and participate in drug and alcohol experimentation, sexual interaction with younger and/or older participants, running away. Because of difficulties with understanding the relationship between cause and effect, teens such as Kristin often are impulsive, which can lead to poor decisions. When questioned about her choices to engage in sexual relationships with older men, Kristin would acknowledge remorse for decisions she was making, but was unable to make the same connection at the time the situation or choice was presenting itself. Unfortunately, the inability to understand cause and effect is easily linked to a lack of awareness of social cues. Often children and adolescents with FASDs misread social cues from their peers and will then proceed to engage in inappropriate gestures, words, and behaviors without realizing the social ramifications.

Developmentally, adolescents have their emotional, physical and social plate full. The flood of hormones and body changes influence adolescents and their behaviors in most of their actions throughout the day. Further, adding the component of prenatal alcohol exposure and the associated changes within the brain complicates the developmental phase of adolescence even more. Natalie Novick reports in her article, *FAS: Preventing and*

Treating Sexual Deviancy that inappropriate sexual behavior is one of the most prevalent secondary disabilities of FAS and ARND.[2]

SEXUAL DEVELOPMENT

As we delve into issues of sexuality in adolescents with FASDs, understanding basic sexual development is important. Below is a description of the sexual development phases from infancy to adulthood for children and adolescents *not* prenatally exposed to alcohol and/or illicit drugs.

Infant to 3 years old

Babies and toddlers are constantly learning during the first three years of their lives. They are discovering and are naturally curious about their own and others' bodies. At this stage, toddlers will repeat what they have learned. If body parts are given a name, whether anatomically correct or slang, they will repeat the words with little or no inhibition. Infants and toddlers may experience sexual responses such as vaginal lubrication or an erection.

Children 4 to 5 years old

During this phase of sexual development, the child may continue to experience vaginal lubrication or an erection. Four- and five-year olds tend to be more curious about their bodies and the differences between male and female, and may explore those differences through play. There will be more touching of their own genitals. Traditional roles are starting to be recognized, and this is the phase in which a "million" questions are asked, most usually, "Why?" This is a time to teach the child how babies are made using the clinical terms for the body parts and how the baby winds up in the uterus.

Children 6 to 8 years old

During this developmental phase children tend to stay within their own gender to find friends. If we think back to the schoolyard, first and second graders are segregated for the most part by gender. Understanding gender differences is more pronounced, and there is a stigma associated with crossing the gender line, which often includes teasing at this age. There may be some same gender experimentation at this age.

It is at this age that children begin to better understand the attitudes and values concerning sexuality of those around them and may become less likely to ask questions based on the caregiver's attitude toward the subject. By this time, children have developed a stronger self- image as it relates not only to their gender but also their body image and may look to the media, movies, peers, and other sources to learn more about sex.

Children 9 to 12
In this age range, children understand more and more who they are as young people, their own sexuality and thoughts of how they will express it. Our pre-teens are very conscientious of their bodies and are wondering if they are "normal." They will wonder if masturbating or having erotic dreams is typical. Continuing education and dialogue during this phase offers opportunities to continue building the stage for appropriate expression of sexual behavior. Having conversations regarding the child's current development also provides those moments to continue to teach about puberty and further changes and developments to the body.

Children may be quite touchy during this phase concerning conversations about sexuality and may mask their anxiety by expressing that they already know the information. As we can determine through the previous developmental phases, the relationship between the caregiver and the child is critical in developing the safe and trusting relationship necessary for having these conversations.

Children at this age understand sexual jokes and innuendos and value privacy a great deal. Parents often are surprised they are no longer welcome in the bathroom while the pre-teen is bathing, and the days of running around the house naked are more than likely gone.

Children 13 to 17 years old
Early adolescents and adolescents are keenly aware of their changing bodies but may be less aware of their heightened emotional changes. They understand they are sexual and are becoming involved in knowing and recognizing

what healthy and unhealthy relationships look like. Teens may engage in sexual acts that may or may not include sexual intercourse. There is a clarity that occurs for most teens that includes understanding in concrete terms the ramifications of sexual intercourse, such as sexually transmitted diseases and pregnancy.

Teens are capable of engaging in conversations and learning about committed, loving relationships. As parents, involving teens in these conversations and normalizing their questions and thoughts will enhance their ability to make appropriate decisions when it comes to participating in sexual behaviors. It is during this phase that teens become more aware and understand their own sexual orientation.

Children 18 years and older
As young adults, many will enter into intimate sexual, emotional relationships. Most young adults are certain of their sexual orientation but still may explore other sexual behaviors. They begin to understand more clearly long term planning for committed relationships and how their sexual behavior plays a part in this. Many will begin to focus on others, as opposed to their world centering on themselves.

For most children and adolescents regardless of prenatal exposure to alcohol, sexual development follows these phases. The concerns for children and adolescents with FASDs are primarily related to the young person's developmental age not coinciding with his or her chronological age. The teen is developing sexually but may not have the cognitive capabilities to appropriately manage the changes emotionally and physically. The diminished ability for children and adolescents with FASDs to identify social cues, make safe and healthy decisions, and read facial and body expressions may lead to inappropriate sexual behavior. Adolescents with FASDs may misread a smile, a comment, and/or an act of kindness as a sexual invitation. This places these children and adolescents at a greater risk of being exploited or committing sexual offenses due to their lack of awareness and understanding of age appropriate boundaries and acceptable sexual gestures and behaviors. As in the case of Kristin, teens with FASDs can easily become convinced that they are "loved" by an exploitive older person and would do anything asked of them.

Social media and exposure to material with sexual content may provide subtle, or not so subtle, hints relating to sexual behaviors the adolescent with FASDs is incapable of processing appropriately. For instance, viewing pornographic material may heighten the sexual response in the adolescent with FASDs and encourage him or her to act solely on the physical responses without using proper decision-making. Freier indicates that there are significant effects that sexually explicit materials have on children. First, since children imitate what they see as part of their natural development and since they often tell children whom they have power over what to do, there is an increased danger for children exposed to pornographic material to sexually abuse other children. Constant exposure of young children to child pornography can result in imitation or buildup of emotional tension that may or may not find release by action. This can result in harmful acts toward another child[3]. In addition, movies, television, and video games with sexually explicit material may lead the impaired adolescent to act inappropriately. Having limited ability to process the explicit information appropriately may cause the adolescent to imitate the behavior, believing it is allowed.

EXTERNAL BRAIN

When addressing sexual development and behavior in teens with FASDs and strategies to guide and protect them, the concept of an "external brain" becomes especially important. Dr. Sterling Clarren, a pioneer in the field of FAS research and clinical care, first developed the term "external brain." The "external brain" refers to the presence of another responsible person (parent, teacher, job coach, sibling) who can mentor, assist, guide, supervise, and/or support the affected person to maximize success (which may need to be redefined as the avoidance of addiction, arrest, unwanted pregnancy, homelessness, or accidental death).[4] The "external brain" is the people and relationships in the child's life that operate in the ways of a mentor, giving guidance and assistance to decision-making and helping process the events that may be occurring in the adolescent's life.

Educating caregivers as to the importance of the "external brain" has a significant role in assisting children and adolescents in making safe and healthy decisions related to their sexual behavior. Building a support system of "external brains" within the adolescent's life reduces the opportunities for the teen to respond and/or make decisions that may place himself or others in jeopardy. Chasnoff shares in his book, *The Mystery of Risk,* that the external brain basically teaches the child strategies for organizing, planning and completing a task – the higher order executive functioning skills.[5] The ongoing teaching, repetition, and development of these skills are crucial to the adolescent's development of cognitive, social, and emotional functioning.

Involving responsible people who have positive, healthy relationships with the adolescent will help support the teen's daily decisions. These partners also can provide assistance and respite to the parents in the supervision of the child. This supportive network acts as a "protective web" around the child. The act of developing and educating the people who will be "external brains" in the child's life takes consistency and commitment on the part of the parent and the support person. Involving and educating teachers, siblings, pastor and/or coach in understanding the impact of FASDs on the child's development and giving them guidelines in assisting the adolescent, will provide opportunities to incorporate "external brains" from a variety of directions in the child's life.

Most often in normal adolescent development, the teen will seek guidance from those around her other than the parent. As we know, most adolescents' focus is their social life and the friends surrounding them. The same will be true for children with FASDs. Ensuring that the proper people are the "external brain" and that they have the skills, education, and motivation to assist the child in healthy ways is *critically* important. The community of support and care in having multiple "external brains" across the span of childhood and adolescence, and often into adulthood, will offer the greatest possibility for success.

WHAT PARENTS SHOULD KNOW ABOUT SEX EDUCATION FOR YOUTH WITH FASDs

Early intervention always is a key to addressing concerns. This especially holds true with sex education for adolescents with FASDs. Regrettably, intervention in these circumstances necessarily is an ongoing process because the damage to judgment and decision-making caused by prenatal alcohol exposure is permanent. Education and repetition of appropriate social skills and boundaries with the identification of danger as early as possible may aid in changing the trajectory of the adolescent's sexual decisions and behaviors. This starts with the caregivers' fully understanding typical sexual development and expressing their personal value system regarding sexual behavior. As adults, our own upbringing, sexual development, and expression will influence how we raise our own children. In addition, religion, spirituality, and experiences in our internal family structure and external influences will guide how we interact with our child about his or her sexual development.

Caregivers must always be aware of their child's friends and relationships in order to assist in preventing inappropriate sexual behaviors (this applies to typical teens and those with FASDs). As caregivers, we must work through our own discomfort of having these delicate conversations with our children and teens. If we do not discuss sexuality and sexual behaviors with the adolescent, the young person most definitely will seek information from others who may not have the same value system as the caregiver or the best interest of the child at heart.

All humans are sexual beings. Appropriate sexual development stems from providing appropriate socialization skills that must be taught from an early age. Based on the limitations of a brain impaired by prenatal exposure to alcohol, the constant training and teaching of the reasons why, what, when, where, and how things are approached is critical.[3] For the child who has not yet begun to explore his or her sexuality, parents have an advantage. The best way to prevent inappropriate sexual touching is to give the child guidelines and coping skills he or she can use when faced with a desire to make physical contact with another person.[5] The teaching of sexuality and appropriate sexual behavior to children and adolescents promotes healthy attitudes regarding sex. This also builds self-esteem and a comfort level in knowing they can have open and honest conversations related to a growing curiosity regarding their own development. In addition, it provides opportunities to build skills while promoting the value system and expected behaviors or goals for the teen.

It is especially important for caregivers, teachers, and medical professionals to interact with children and adolescents with FASDs at the youth's developmental level. Ignoring the adolescent's sexual development is not the answer. Presenting information and educating the child or teen at his individual intellectual ability is essential in keeping them and others safe. The information presented to the child and/or teen must be concrete. Going back to the use of why, what, when, where, and how things are approached is critical to providing consistent learning in various situations.

FASDs AND INAPPROPRIATE SEXUAL BEHAVIOR

Early diagnosis, treatment, and educating caregivers may assist in changing the trajectory of adolescents with FASDs. O'Conner and Paley indicate that the identification and the provision of specific treatments to address unique features of this developmental disability are critical since early identification and treatment have been demonstrated to be protective against more serious secondary disabilities.[6]

In reviewing the literature on sexuality among adolescents diagnosed with FASDs, many of the same issues arise regarding inappropriate sexual behaviors. Oftentimes the adolescent does not demonstrate effective boundaries with others including honoring personal space and/or making sexual advances to the point of touching another person without permission. There also is the danger of the young person's engaging in activities that may exploit the teen. Although extreme deviant sexual behaviors occur in a very small percentage of youth with FASDs, the risk remains high for all youth affected by prenatal exposure to alcohol: promiscuity that can place the adolescent in danger of a sexually transmitted disease (STD) and unwanted pregnancy, voyeuristic behaviors, masturbation in public, indecent exposure, incest, and unusual sexual behavior that may include paraphilic behaviors such as pedophilia, zoophilia, sexual sadism, and exhibitionism.[7]

An additional risk for all youth in our society today is the ever-growing access to instant technology. The use of cell phones, texting, sexting, sending nude photographs, and internet access make it difficult for a teen with impaired brain functioning and impulsive actions to process appropriate behaviors when others around him or her may not be doing the same.

WHAT DO WE DO?

The single most important intervention children and teens with FASDs need is a healthy, positive, loving, nurturing relationship with a caregiver. Providing avenues of connectedness for the child or teen in relation to his family, community, and school increases the opportunities for the youth to engage in appropriate activities. Based on powerful and positive relationships, a child's self-esteem is developed and encouraged as he matures. On the other hand, a good deal of the research indicates that attachment between caregiver and the child with FASDs is a significant area of concern and struggle for parents. Therapy with a mental health specialist who has expertise in the area of FASDs and attachment becomes a must at the first sign of a disconnection.

In regard to early intervention, there are some recommendations that might guide parents and caregivers in addressing sexuality in children with FASDs:[8]

- Use clear, simple, and concrete rules about sexuality and repeat them over and over.
- Teach children to ask permission before touching others.
- Teach children about personal space. Because sensory processing deficits do not allow children affected by prenatal alcohol exposure to judge a socially acceptable distance, provide a concrete guide to talking with others, such as everyone has to be an arm's length away.
- Don't talk to strangers.
- Teach and repeat that unprotected sex is never safe.
- Masturbation is done only in private, in your bedroom, at home.

- Talk about sex and sexuality–often, repeatedly.
- Role-play appropriate behaviors:
  - how to hug and touch others appropriately
  - how to ask someone out on a date
  - how to say no to sexual advances.
- Encourage group dating.
- Provide a concrete strategy of how to get "out" of a situation and whom to contact.
- Supervise your child–no matter the age.

Based on sexual development as it occurs in typically developing children, we can identify ways to promote healthy sexual development. Although this chapter focuses on children and adolescents with FASDs, it is important to know effective strategies to increase healthy sexual development in all children. Through each developmental phase, suggestions are provided for families to further healthy sexual development for their children.

SEXUAL DEVELOPMENT - HOW TO EDUCATE[8]
Infant to 3 years old
As caregivers we must be mindful of our own views, thoughts, and values system when teaching sexual development and must avoid making children feel guilty, embarrassed, or ashamed of their body parts. There are so many opportunities during this phase of development to appropriately touch a child, build trust, and begin the positive modeling for healthy sexual development. One of the responsibilities of the caregiver is to help infants and toddlers feel good about their bodies. Teaching the names of body parts early on in the child's development helps to normalize the identification of the genital areas and creates a natural, healthy attitude toward sexuality. Much of the research recommends the use of clinical names when teaching toddlers the genital areas. Teaching the anatomical differences is important in the development of children. It is equally important for toddlers to know that they may say no at any time to unwanted touch. Begin teaching what the words private and respect mean. Also, caregivers may

have opportunities during this phase to point to a woman who is pregnant and in very simple terms explain "a baby is growing."

Children 4 to 5 years old
Teach children at this age about privacy and appropriate places to talk about sexuality and that the home is the place they can touch their genitals. Continuing to teach appropriate names of the genitals will reinforce earlier learning. Also, implanting the trust in children at this age that they can talk to you about anything, including sexuality, begins to set the stage for many more conversations as they develop.

Children 6 to 8 years old
Parents may feel a sense of relief in this phase because children are asking fewer questions, but this is a critical time for parents to continue teaching about sexuality. Fewer questions do not mean less curiosity. We want our children to learn about sexuality from us. Continue to offer open dialogue regarding the child's own sexuality, as well as the differences in the make-up of families (i.e., same sex parents, single parents, divorced families, and blended families). This age also is a time to begin teaching basics to children about love and relationships and, in very simple terms, sexual abuse and the importance of saying "no" when they are uncomfortable.

Preparing children during this time for puberty and the transformation that will occur assists children in being ready for the developmental changes. Children typically handle change in an easier fashion when they are prepared. Children are entering puberty earlier and earlier, although most will not begin to have bodily changes during this developmental phase.

Children 9 to 12
It is important to continue teaching children at this age that their body functions and changes are normal, natural, and healthy. Continuing to prepare them for puberty and ongoing changes will decrease anxiety. Respecting our children's right to privacy is important, but privacy does not mean isolation. It is imperative that caregivers continue open, honest, healthy

discussions as children begin the approach to puberty. We must assist children in understanding that the rate in which people develop differs from person to person. Often children at this age will compare themselves to their peers as far as height and weight are concerned.

Having open conversations at this stage regarding intercourse, sexually transmitted diseases, and pregnancy is important in preparing children to understand they have much more cognitive and emotional growth ahead of them. It is important to discuss the detrimental behavior of engaging in sexual activities at this age in terms of their physical and emotional health and social unacceptability of this choice. Explain to children that abstinence is healthy and natural at this age and as they mature they will become more prepared for sexual engagement in various forms and not necessarily sexual intercourse. It is necessary to explain to children the differences and the relationship between sexual and emotional feelings. There may be children at this age who will be curious about contraception. As a caregiver, being open to the conversation continues to provide a safe place for the child to learn more and the caregiver to stay involved in the child's cognitive understanding of her sexual development.

Children 13 to 17 years old
Throughout the previous phases and continuing into this phase of sexual development it is important that the family's values and religious thoughts are a part of the conversation regarding sexual behavior and, specifically, intercourse. Communicate with teens the importance of waiting to engage in sexual behaviors. Acknowledge that sex is pleasurable but make clear that it is most enjoyable when initiated within a committed, loving, mature relationship. Describe to teens how to have a healthy relationship with another person and how to express love and closeness without becoming sexually intimate. This includes how to talk and get to know one another, holding hands, kissing, writing notes.

Parents must be clear in their expectations of appropriate sexual behaviors within the context of the family's value system. The expectations a teen must consider prior to participating in sexual behaviors should include at what age it is appropriate, mutual consent is always a must, contraceptive use and options, and how to express love and intimacy. Caregivers should express to teens the importance of knowing their own level of self-control and their ability to make good decisions in the "thick" of things. Talking through possible scenarios assists teens in having a plan if a situation becomes too intimate. Knowing how to stop and how to use their words in communicating the desire to stop is equally important. Teaching clear verbal replies to unwanted sexual advances may keep the teen from engaging further in sexual behaviors.

A part of the conversation that must occur is the reality of risk for pregnancy or an STD if a teen chooses to engage in sexual behavior. If this happens, the teen must know what to do. As far as pregnancy the teen should know the options available. There is the choice to parent the baby, abort, or place the baby for adoption. If a teen believes he or she has a STD, you and the teen must discuss the available options. The teen may come to you or see their doctor with their concerns but it is imperative that they know to never ignore the signs of an STD. Discussing with teens the need to keep them safe and sexually healthy includes teaching them that sexting, sending nude photos, and explicit sexual talk could be damaging and exploitive beyond the relationship they are currently in.

Children 18 years and older
Accepting that our children are now young adults is important in their overall development. As we have prepared our children through the development phases, we need to continue to allow the ability to openly communicate and seek answers to their questions as young adults. Respecting our children as adults and encouraging them with good decision- making while communicating with them the responsibilities that accompany the choices is critical in continuing to have healthy communication.

For the child/teen with FASDs, interventions and teachable moments appear much the same as for the typically developing child. The caregiver will need more of an emphasis on the information to be presented to the child in a developmentally appropriate manner with multiple repetitions, constant supervision, and continuous support and guidance. Suggestions for interventions and teachable moments include:[9]

- Talk about sexuality even if it is uncomfortable. If the young person does not get information from the parent, he or she will get it from someone else.
- Teach and practice to always ask for permission before touching.
- Practice touching others appropriate and respectful manner, such as shaking hands and hugging.
- Use language that is clear and simple when talking about sex. Use the appropriate name for sexual acts and body parts to avoid confusion.
- The "external brain" is important. Supervision, by a trusted friend or family member, cousin or sibling could double date or even go on practice dates.
- Know where, and with whom the teens are going out. Ensure an "external brain" is in the group. Encourage young couples to attend family events, meet up with friends or get involved in community activities. Let others know providing extra supervision at events like school dances or camping trips is crucial.
- Know what is being taught at school regarding sexuality and ensure that the school reinforces what is being taught at home.
- Teach how to ask someone out on a date or how to say not to sexual advances. Role playing can be very useful.
- Make any rules about sexuality simple, consistent, absolute, and concrete.
- Demonstrate use of birth control methods and show what birth control looks like.

CONTINUUM OF CARE

The questions remain. What do we do with the adolescent who is exhibiting high-risk sexual behaviors? How do caregivers manage these situations and protect the young person with FASDs? Interventions for people with FASDs transitioning into adulthood are critical because substance use and abuse problems, high-risk sexual behavior, and illegal activities may emerge or worsen during this developmental period.[10]

Due to the high risk for adolescents becoming involved in situations and activities that place them and others in jeopardy, the engagement of mental health professionals is necessary. At the first indication of concern, caregivers are encouraged to engage external supports. Treatment interventions may vary based on the most prevalent issues presented to the clinician but the engagement of an outside source may assist the adolescent's ability to be open and willing to learn based on the new relationship. The treatment goals developed between the therapist and the teen often will address the high-risk actions. Discussions may center on how to increase and improve the teen's abilities to make better decisions; concrete steps in how to solve problems (such as a Decision Tree); strategies for regulating their own behaviors (such as *How Does Your Engine Run*®)[11]; and how to control sexual impulses, especially in social situations. Teaching teens with FASDs how to self-talk to assist with the retrieval of information is important in reminding them of appropriate actions. Receiving input from their "external brains" that offer cues to appropriate responses and offer feedback of how a situation might be handled differently may promote increased development. Adolescents with FASDs respond best to "common sense" education. The use of visual and experiential activities will engage the teen for a longer period of time and will offer cues that will assist the young person in recovering the information. It is important for providers and caregivers to remember the use of lecture or control tactics rarely is effective with most people, let alone children and adolescents with FASDs. The treatment provider who is working with adolescents with FASDs will need to reassess the treatment strategies frequently to assure the teen is continuing to learn and apply the skills in daily living. When strategies are not effective, the provider must adjust the approach and meet the child at a point and in a way that the young person is able to grasp the concepts, to practice, and to implement the skills.

Treatment interventions must include educating the caregiver and processing with the caregiver what the adolescent with FASDs is experiencing. Involving the entire family in treatment is an excellent option as well. It will provide understanding for all and not classify the adolescent with FASDs as the identified patient. Treatment then becomes an opportunity for the family as a whole to develop strategies that assist one another. Developing the relationship between the caregiver, family and the teen is essential to the development of open communication and provides the foundation for having difficult, sensitive conversations in the future.

INTENSIVE SERVICES

Intensive services may be approached in several ways.
- Increase the frequency of family mental health services. Instead of services one time a week, increase services to 3 or 4 times a week until the family and teen are stable.
- Include services in the home and/or in the school such as therapeutic behavioral services (TBS), children's intensive services (CIS), or wrap-around services. These services are typically provided several times a week and for a lengthy period of time during each intervention. The length of time can be from two to four hours a day. The advantage to implementing these services on-site is they offer caregivers and teachers opportunities to learn through the treatment provider modeling the appropriate responses and interventions when the teen is expressing undesirable behaviors.

There are times the adolescent exhibiting high-risk sexual behaviors may need additional supports beyond what the caregiver and the provider may be able to offer. In order to assure the teen's safety, he may require a short-term placement in a residential treatment center in order to receive 24-hour supervision and intensive mental health services. In extreme cases, the adolescent that presents as a danger to self and/or others may require a short-term placement in a psychiatric hospital in order to receive 24-hour supervision and intensive mental health services.

CONCLUSION

Whatever happened to Kristin? Kristin and her parents began intensive mental health treatment services focusing on immediately decreasing the behaviors putting Kristin at risk; increasing communication between the parents and Kristin; seeking a medication evaluation from a psychiatrist; further educating the parents; and identifying, developing and educating "external" brains in Kristin's life.

Intensive services were provided in the home and at the school. Very early in the process the treatment provider learned several things that may have influenced the recent unwanted behaviors. The parents themselves were quite uncomfortable having conversations with Kristin regarding sexual behavior. The treatment provider had several private discussions with Bill and Sue. They focused on finding a balance for them in speaking more freely with Kristin about her sexual development and behaviors. It was also determined that as Kristin was maturing physically, the parents had reverted to their own parent's way of communicating which was mostly lecture and control. A review of the skills learned in therapy and adapting the skills to apply to their teen assisted Bill and Sue in communicating with Kristin in a more productive manner. One of the key findings was that Kristin had previously been home-schooled and only recently entered public school. Kristin was overwhelmed with the stimulation around her, the access to so many other people, and the expectations for her success. Setting boundaries with Kristin and having her model the behaviors expected along with educating the school staff to assist with being her "external brain" allowed Kristin to improve her behavior drastically. The use of a "code word" in the classroom assisted Kristin, without embarrassment, in stopping an unwanted behavior without drawing attention specifically to her. Kristin and her parents developed a list of people whom Kristin identified as caring about her and wanting what was best for her. They discussed how they would engage these people in learning about her impairment and how this group could support her.

Intensive services occurred for six months in the home and school, but it was not always smooth, nor easy. The family worked very hard to change their interaction in order to keep their daughter safe. Kristin continues to require the "external brains" in her life and her parents continue to monitor her activities and relationships very closely.

NOTES

1. O'Connor MJ, Paley B. Psychiatric Conditions Associated with Prenatal Alcohol Exposure, *Developmental Disabilities Research Reviews* 2009;15:225-234.

2. Novick N. "FAS: Preventing and Treating Sexual Deviancy." *The Challenge of Fetal Alcohol Syndrome: Overcoming Secondary Disabilities* (162-170), University of Washington Press, Seattle, 1997.

3. Babikian T, Freier, MC. "Sexuality and Society", In Helm, H. W., Jr., & McBride, D. C., *Many Voices: An Introduction to Social Issues* (pp. 172-199). Berrien Springs, MI: Andrews University Press, 2006

4. Teresa Kellerman, *The External Brain*, 2003.

5. Chasnoff IJ, *The Mystery of Risk,* NTI Upstream, Chicago, 2010.

6. O'Connor MJ, Paley B. Psychiatric Conditions Associated with Prenatal Alcohol Exposure, *Developmental Disabilities Research Reviews* 2009;15: 225-234.

7. Streissguth et al 2004, Risk Factors for Adverse Life Outcomes in Fetal Alcohol Syndrome and Fetal Alcohol Effects.

8. Fetal Alcohol Spectrum Disorders – Relationships and Sexuality – www.fasdwaterlooregion.ca/strategies-tools/relatioships-and-sexuality.

9. FASD Support Network of Saskatchewan, "FASDs Tips for Parents and Caregivers: Numbers 1 - 20".

10. Paley B, O'Conner MJ. Behavioral Interventions for Children and Adolescents with Fetal Alcohol Spectrum Disorders, *Alcohol Research & Health,* 34(1).

11. TherapyWorks, Inc.; www.alertprogram.com.

CHAPTER 5 *Parenting*

S.O.S: A PARENT'S CRY FOR HELP OR A SURVIVAL STRATEGY?

Carole Hurley, J.D.

Carole Hurley, an administrate law judge in Texas, offers a first-person glimpse into her life raising her adoptive daughter Kara through adolescence and into young adulthood. This unique chapter is a behind-the-scenes look at how together they cope with the young lady's neurocognitive difficulties caused by her prenatal exposure to alcohol. Ms. Hurley explains why structure, routine, and repetition are so crucial to raising an adolescent with FASDs.

Depending on the day, my S.O.S can be either a cry for help or a term I use as my strategy to survive. When it is a cry for help there aren't too many people who know how to respond. They haven't lived with the challenges my family lives with daily, and frankly some of them are taken aback and a little frightened by us. As a survival strategy, S.O.S. stands for Structure, Organization, and Supervision. These three tactics have guided me as I raise my precious but challenging children.

I am the mother of two daughters whose birth mothers drank during their pregnancies. My older daughter, Kara, is twenty and my younger is eleven. Raising Kara to chronological adulthood has brought my greatest pleasure and my greatest pain. I use the term "chronological adulthood" for the reason that the law and society see her as an adult because she is over eighteen years old. Developmentally she is closer to fourteen and far from an adult. The choices Kara makes, her lack of judgment, and her inability to foresee natural consequences are all about six years behind her chronological age. Well-meaning friends constantly tell me that all teenagers are immature, don't anticipate consequences, and make poor decisions… but those "typical" teenagers learn from their experiences, and by the time they are twenty they are able to manage far more of life's challenges than my child can.

I often use humor as a stress reliever, and I recommend that families grappling with raising a child with challenges try to see the humor in situations when they can. Laughter is healthy, and recognizing the absurdity of our experiences and finding a nugget of humor in them can lighten the weight of our worry and fear. When my children see that I am able to laugh about an incident, they learn that being different isn't the end of the world. Parents of those "typical" children sometimes think I am insensitive, but I am just searching for the bright side of our daily struggles. As my younger daughter told me when she was 6: "I'm so glad I'm not a 'typical kid' Mom. Those kids are so boring!" There are plenty of times that the issues we face are no laughing matter, so when you can, laugh with your children about the crazy lives you all are living.

STRUCTURE

When Kara first came to live with me, in the back of my mind I knew she was a little different, but since she was my dream come true, I didn't give it much thought. I was in my late thirties and had some pretty definite ideas about child rearing after spending years watching those around me practice their parenting techniques. As it turned out, starting my family later and having the chance to sit back and observe others benefited my daughters and me immensely, although looking back now I realize that at the time I had no idea what I was doing! But I trusted my gut and knew that a lot of structure was what they needed. I don't see how I could have possibly parented my children if I had been younger, with less life experience and less time watching and learning.

Like so many adoptive parents, when Kara came to me I knew nothing about prenatal alcohol exposure and was just relieved that my child's biological mom didn't have the money to use drugs. Bio-mom spent a lot of time on the streets, so alcohol was readily available, and she used it like everyone else around her. It never occurred to me that her alcohol use would be an issue that would shape the rest of my life, my career, and most importantly, the life of my beautiful, perfect, little girl.

From the day Kara arrived I put a careful structure in place in our home. As a single parent with a busy and challenging professional career I had to manage my time well, both at work and at home. We lived a very structured life: Kara got up, got dressed, and ate breakfast at the same time in the same order every day. Every evening at 6:30 I bathed her, washed her hair, put on her jammies, brushed her teeth, rocked her for ten minutes, put on the same lullaby CD, and turned out the light. Every weekday was the same, and although on weekends we had free time, we still got up, got dressed, ate meals, and went to bed on the same schedule.

During those early childhood years I kept an overnight bag in the trunk of my car with everything for a bath, pajamas, and a change of clothing, along with a *Pack 'n Play*. If we were at a friend's house in the evening, at 6:30 we went through our routine and I put her down in a quiet bedroom. I have a picture of Kara at age 6 taking her afternoon nap on a bench at Disney World. Now **that** is structure! And structure is what Kara thrived on.

Everything in Kara's closet was appropriate for daycare or school. All of her socks were identical. All of her t-shirts went with all of her shorts and pants. All of her shoes were acceptable to wear to school. Although I selected her clothing each morning, if she had chosen her own there would not have been any arguments. When every choice is a good choice everyone wins. Another benefit of having all of the socks (and panties) identical is that a child with sensory issues or compulsion challenges doesn't have the stress of putting on socks or underwear that doesn't feel right. It all feels the same and looks the same. That means one less thing to struggle over in the morning.

We generally have the same thing for breakfast every school day. I mean EVERY school day. For the past 17 years. I have no ability to control or change what happened to their brains, but I can control what goes into their bodies when they are with me. Every morning I make them a simple hot breakfast. They like it, they don't have any sensory issues with the texture or taste, and I feel like I have done one thing that might help them as they start their day. Our children work twice as hard as "typical" children to manage their behavior and master the school curriculum each day, so if I can get them out the door without a meltdown I feel like I have done a good job.

My children don't do well with noise or transition so riding the school bus has never been a good idea. I drive them to school and pick them up each day. Traditional after-school programs are too noisy and chaotic for them, so they have always either come home right after school or gone to a small in-home after-school program. Managing their sensory input is critical to their being able to control their behavior. The schools they have attended have not always recognized this, so it is my job to anticipate problems and resolve them before anything happens.

From pre-kindergarten at the age of 3 years through kindergarten, Kara attended a private church school. The uniform and the natural structure of the curriculum were perfect for her. She always knew what was going to happen next, and there was little spontaneity. While I wished she could enjoy the creative atmosphere of a Montessori program, I felt in my heart it just wasn't for Kara. Little did I know at the time how right I was. If Kara had been given the freedom to choose what to do in a classroom it would have been a disaster. She either wouldn't have done anything or she would have only participated in one activity and probably convinced the rest of the class to do only what she was doing.

I have friends who live for spontaneity. At a moment's notice they pack into the car and go do something fun. My children do not do that. If I could even get them into the car that quickly for some unplanned fun event someone would be screaming before we got out of the driveway! Even a spur of the moment trip to the grocery store can spell disaster. Daily my eleven-year old asks, "What's the plan?" It doesn't matter if the plan is the same it has been for nearly every day of her life. She likes to hear me say exactly what she already knows the plan is.

Kara has always been very sure of herself, especially when she is wrong. When she was young other children were drawn to that sense of confidence and certainty, and would follow her and do what she told them to do. What was really happening in Kara's brain was that when she had a thought or an idea it never went any further. It never crossed her mind that she could be wrong or that there could be any other way of thinking, so she was always confident. Because she never learned from the times she actually was wrong, her confidence in herself was never shaken. However, as she got older that sureness was no longer an asset. In eleventh grade when Kara made an A on her first three Spanish tests she was sure she knew the subject, and quit doing the homework and quit studying. Imagine her dismay when she failed the fourth test. But true to form, once she believed she knew the material she refused to study and failed the next few tests.

At age 4 my equally confident younger daughter, who does not speak Spanish, actually convinced a bi-lingual child in her class that she was fluent in Spanish and that his parents had taught him wrong. She was so sure that she *was* speaking Spanish that he, and the other children, believed her. She also believed she could fly, and that caused another host of issues, at home, at school, and out in public. I kept her away from staircases and high furniture as much as possible in those days.

Like many of our children with prenatal alcohol exposure, Kara has a superior I.Q., and when she will cooperate with the structure required to do homework, turn it in, and study for tests effectively, she can make high grades. She was on the A – B honor roll her freshman and sophomore years in high school. It required a great deal of effort to keep her engaged in the work to make those grades, but she and I both put in the effort and it paid off.

As the curriculum grew more complex and her willingness to cooperate dropped, she began to struggle, and our relationship became strained. By the time Kara was a high school junior, teachers and administrators expected her to know the school routine and independently have the skills to be academically successful. After all, she was engaging, cute, and smart. Realistically, however, she was developmentally closer to a middle-school student. When she wrote assignments in her planner she wouldn't remember that she had. She was so sure of herself that when I asked her each afternoon if she had homework she would say "no." Since she didn't remember that she had an assignment or that she had written it down, it never occurred to her that she could have forgotten that she had one, and it would not occur to her to look at her planner to see. Typical of a seventh or eighth grader she didn't want to do homework, she didn't want to cooperate with anyone in charge, including me, and she didn't have the insight to understand the consequences. That is an example of the issue of developmental versus chronological age faced by so many families. Her behavior would probably be okay in seventh or eighth grade; colleges don't look at middle-school grades. But by eleventh grade our children are expected to have passed those developmental milestones and to be preparing for their future. High schools aren't equipped to support our children, especially when they have average or above intelligence.

As a parent I struggled to help teachers and school administrators understand that Kara was only doing what Kara could do. Her damaged brain did not allow for her to use another approach or even recognize her flawed process. She didn't purposefully fail to write in her planner, or think to look in it after school, or study for tests. Her damaged brain lacked the capacity to even comprehend that what she did on any given day impacted tomorrow or next week or next year.

By the time Kara was nine or ten I realized that the everyday tasks most of us perform without thinking: brush our teeth, wash our face, take our medications, lock the front door on the way out…*close the front door on the way out*…just weren't engrained in Kara's thought process. In spite of well-meaning friends trying to convince me, "All teenagers are like that," this was *not* like "all teenagers."

To help her with the structure of those basic tasks we started using checklists. A typical morning checklist included: brush hair, brush teeth, wash face, put on deodorant, dress, eat breakfast, unload dishwasher, feed dog, give dog water, check backpack, go to school. After a few years she began to balk at the idea of using checklists – she knew other kids her age did not need them. So I had her develop her own checklist. That worked for a while, but by the time she was a senior in high school she refused to use checklists, and often the dog went without food, or maybe had no water. Even though every time she fed the dog she also had to give him water she never connected the two tasks. (Not one single time in 15 years of owning a dog did she give him food and water without being reminded to do each task.) She usually brushed her hair, but often forgot to brush her teeth. While she always managed to get all of her clothes on, they were not always clean. One summer when she was 17, she wore the same clothes every day for two weeks…and summers are very hot where we live. (She was terribly insulted when I told her she smelled bad, and insisted that I was just being judgmental.) At least she knows how to make and use checklists and can rely on them if she ever decides they will be helpful.

As Kara became a teenager, structure became even more important in our home. As her peers were beginning to try out independence and make choices about how to spend their time and when to do homework and chores, Kara didn't have the ability to successfully navigate that freedom. We continued to have meals at the same time, go to bed at the same time, and wake up at the same time. Homework was always done immediately when we arrived home in the evening. Kara would sit down at the table while I made dinner in the adjoining kitchen. I was able to keep an eye on what was happening and keep Kara on task.

Year in and year out, 365 days a year, our days have always looked very much the same. In the summer when other children were still out at 9 o'clock playing as the warm summer evenings closed in, my children were taking their baths and getting tucked into bed. Over school breaks when the other teenagers stayed up all night eating junk food and playing computer games, Kara was at home sleeping. When she had the chance to go to sleepovers she usually chose not to, because she did not like staying up late. By the time she was thirteen she was so accustomed to our routine and structure that she was not comfortable without it.

As Kara got older, invitations for social activities slowed. Since she usually chose not to participate, friends stopped asking. Kara was oblivious. Although at school she was very social and talked to everyone, she never really seemed to notice that her friendships were superficial. This was also the age that the developmental differences really began to show and when I had to become much more vigilant about where she went and with whom. Kara's two most significant deficits are that she cannot tell or sense the passage of time and she cannot use money. Those two deficits coupled with her poor decision making jeopardized her safety if she were out with other teenagers.

I deal with protecting my children from situations they are not ready to handle by keeping our family very busy with interesting activities that the two girls don't want to miss out on. It is exhausting, but they are too busy to notice what other children are doing to feel bad that they are left out. Kara danced classical Russian ballet until she was fourteen, which meant three intense ballet classes each week, and an additional class every Saturday in the spring. When she quit ballet she picked up lacrosse and practiced after school four days a week and had games on Saturdays. Every Friday night was family game night or family movie night. We would work together in the kitchen to make homemade pizza and then settle in to watch a Netflix movie or play board games. I have played so much Scrabble and Monopoly that I want to scream! We went camping, traveled to see friends and family members in other states, went to museums, hiked, volunteered for community service projects, and built family traditions and memories that I hope will help my daughters feel connected and grounded as they grow into adulthood. I worry that because Kara has such poor short-term memory, once she leaves our home it may not even occur to her that we developed traditions that she no longer engages in. I believe, though, that creating a tight family unit with a special place for each of them has given my children a sense of belonging to something special. I hope that sense of belonging will help them avoid seeking out a sense of belonging from people who are inappropriate.

Sometimes it is so hard to be calm and patient, and I have my screaming moments when I lose control, but through it all I try to express absolute, unconditional love and acceptance of who my children are. That doesn't mean acceptance of everything they *do*. When they break the serious rules I have to follow through with appropriate consequences, but I try to do so with as much composure as I can manage. My children do much better when I can stay calm in the face of their outbursts and tantrums.

ORGANIZATION

Children and teens with FASDs usually have a hard time getting and staying organized. Along about third grade, teachers expect students to begin keeping track of their materials, writing down assignments, turning in homework, and managing their backpacks. My children sometimes can't find two shoes that match, much less ever grasp organization principles. My children have the desks that look like small burrowing animals are hibernating there. Their backpacks are a jumble of food, crumpled papers, overdue library books, and broken pencils. They never put papers into the expensive zippered binder that the teacher required every child to have. The organization systems that look so promising on the store shelves will never work in my home.

Even now we still struggle with all things organizational, and the disorganization that my children create wherever they go adds to the stress. The more stress they are under, the more poorly they perform. And as their performance spirals out of control, they become less able to organize, increasing the stress, and so the cycle continues.

When Kara was in fourth grade I decided to simplify what I could at home. We began using baskets and bins to keep the toys and art supplies out of sight. At the end of the day when we come home backpacks are immediately hung on hooks in the laundry room and the lunch boxes are taken into the kitchen. The common areas of the house are picked up before going to bed each night. All toys, books, and clothing are picked up from the bedroom at bedtime. Closet doors are kept closed. The dishwasher is turned on every night, even if it is not full, and emptied every morning. Routine, structure, and organization–by keeping the environment as uncluttered as possible, and always putting backpacks and lunch boxes where they belong, my children's brains are free to focus on more important issues, and we don't have the stress of running around in the morning looking for papers, books, binders, or lunch boxes.

Each day during high school when we arrived home I would insist Kara pull out her planner and we would sit down to complete homework. Often we argued, with Kara insisting she had no homework, only to find that she had several assignments written in her planner. What Kara does not remember does not exist to her, so I believe she was genuinely surprised when she discovered she had homework. That is also the time I took care of reading and signing notes and papers that needed my attention for school the next day. My children learned that I really meant it when I said I would not sign papers, review notes from teachers, or dispense money for school activities in the mornings. If it needed my attention, it had to be done the night before. Reducing our morning stress helps us get out the door with fewer incidents, and helps the two girls to start their day on a happy note.

Each morning we stopped before going out the door for one more check: backpack, lunch, notes for the teacher, assignments, deodorant, teeth brushed. And so our days began. By fifth or sixth grade other mothers were whisking out the door with their children, after a few more years even sending them out to drive themselves to school. Not me. Through her fifth year (yes, it took five years) of high school Kara needed assistance if she were going to get everything together she needed. By that last year, even if she had made her lunch the night before, more often than not she left for school without it. When I would remind her to get it out of the fridge she was furious with me for reminding her, but without the reminder it was always left behind.

When Kara entered high school I realized that the typical backpack, which was always a mess, was not the best way to organize a kid with a disorganized brain. I invested in two sturdy messenger style bags. Two, so that mid-year when the first one fell apart she had an identical one to replace it with. (No mid-year surprise of a bag that looked or felt different.) For each subject I gave her a 1/2-inch white binder. On its spine with a black Sharpie she printed the subject in large easy to read letters. Inside the front cover of the binder she placed two see-through, different colored, three-hole punched poly pockets. With the black Sharpie she printed "Turn in" on the first and "Homework" on the second. They needed to be see-through so she could see if anything was in them. They needed to be colored because the clear ones "disappeared." They needed to be different colors so she could tell that which one she was looking at.

The challenge was getting Kara to pull out the binder when class started. If she did, she could open it and if there was anything in the first pocket (turn in) she knew to turn it in. When a paper was handed out to complete for homework she would put it in the "homework" pocket. In the evening when she pulled out each binder she could readily see if anything had been handed out for homework and when she completed anything that was to be turned in she placed it in the "turn in" pocket, and it was there when (if) she pulled out the binder in class.

This is not a routine Kara ever mastered on her own. I had to sit down with her every evening and look at her planner, then look at her binders and then monitor her until she completed her assignments. All the way through high school she had to have a teacher who was assigned as her case manager make sure she had written the day's assignments down in her planner and that she had everything she needed to complete her work that evening. Given Kara's delightful personality (when she was not at home) and her high intellect, most teachers did not think she needed such a high level of support, and often failed to provide it. She would have to remind teachers of her accommodations, which understandably she didn't always want to do. I spent a lot of time at her high school tracking down teachers and explaining why my child needed such high levels of support and insisting they provide it.

Lockers can be another organizational nightmare. Kara couldn't remember which hallway her locker was in, the locker number, or the combination to the lock. Trying to find the locker and get into it, remembering what she needed to get out of it, transferring things out of and into her messenger bag, and making it through noisy crowded halls to the next class on time was out of the question. She never used her locker for even one day in high school. She kept all of her textbooks at home, and the classrooms had sets of books as well, so she did not need to transport them back and forth.

Every morning at home Kara loaded everything she needed for the day into her messenger bag, grabbed her lacrosse stick, and away she went. She carried everything (including the lacrosse stick) with her all day. I drove her to school most days, and dropped her off right before classes started. She would have preferred that I take her earlier, but that would have given her too much time to socialize, and her concentration would have been broken before the day even started. Unless she was riding with someone else to lacrosse practice I picked her up as soon as classes let out. Again, too much time to socialize unsupervised would have led to her getting into trouble.

By the time Kara reached her senior year her grades had fallen, and she was not eligible to graduate with our state's high school diploma that allows entry into a four-year college. I give her credit for deciding that was not good enough for her. She decided to stay in school for another year and make up the science and math classes she needed for the diploma she wanted. Her fifth year she only had to go to high school half days and decided to take one class at community college. While that sounds wonderful, it was a challenging period for us.

Naturally Kara does best in a highly structured environment. The school system provided that structure beautifully, but college is not at all structured. There is no bell alerting students to be in class and no hall monitor to make students go into the classroom. Classes are offered at different times of the day, in different buildings, and sometimes on different days. Students are responsible for registering themselves and purchasing the books and materials they need. All of this was contrary to how Kara's brain was wired.

By the time Kara finished high school she had become very uncooperative and did not want to be reminded when she did not have her lunch, or the books and binders she needed, or when and where she needed to be at school. By nineteen she refused to put her things away before going to bed and her room was a mess. Sometimes she wore dirty clothes because she couldn't find clean ones in the tangle of clutter on the floor of her bedroom. Sometimes she wore dirty clothes because they were what she wanted to wear and she didn't care if they weren't clean. As her surroundings became more jumbled so it seemed did other areas of her life. Her grades suffered, her moods worsened, and my happy, sweet little girl became angry, irritable, and very unhappy.

Because she refused to cooperate with my attempts to guide her in organizing and structuring her life there was little I could do to help her. Although this has made me deeply sad, she is an adult and I cannot help her if she refuses to allow me to.

SUPERVISION

Unlike typical children, and contrary to what well-meaning friends and family try to convince us, children and teens with FASDs require constant supervision. As they get older, the need for supervision only becomes greater. My kids can't go hang out at the mall like the other teenagers. They can't be left home alone after school. Their online activity has to be monitored carefully. Their judgment is poor, they are developmentally and emotionally delayed; they are vulnerable and can get themselves into serious trouble.

As a single mother, constant supervision has been hard to manage sometimes. I was fortunate to be able to work from home for seven years so I could take my children to school every morning and pick them up after school each afternoon. Traditional after school programs do not offer the degree of supervision my children need. They expect children to be able to do homework independently, and don't realize that if my children are not intently supervised on the playground they will throw rocks at passing cars.

Early on I set boundaries with my children and stuck to them. No boyfriends until age 16, and even then no unchaperoned outings. Kara was nearly out of high school before she was allowed to go out with a boy in a car. It wasn't always pretty–and she was often quite furious with me, but those boundaries kept her safe and gave her some extra time to mature.

When my children went for the rare play date or sleepover at someone else's house I was that mom who asked if there were guns, if they were locked up, and if there would be adult supervision. In middle and high school I asked about alcohol in the home. Some of the other parents thought I was odd, and I was an embarrassment to my children, but my children were safe and that is what counts. Other children were always welcome in our home, where I could keep an eye on what was going on.

Now that Kara is taking classes at community college she is home unsupervised some afternoons. (I no longer work from home.) I periodically take a late lunch hour to make random drive-bys to be sure she is alone (no boys allowed in the house when I am not home). When I find her breaking the rules I have to increase my vigilance…and call the boy's parents. (Have I said it's not pretty?) In a sense supervision is really all about prevention. Typical children learn from their mistakes. Sometimes that is the only way they learn. My children do not learn from their mistakes, so to keep them safe and out of trouble I have to do all I can to prevent their getting into trouble. And supervision is a huge part of prevention.

Raising these daughters of mine has been the most challenging, difficult, beautiful work I have ever done. It remains to be seen how things turn out in the end, but for now everyone is safe. At a stage where most parents are breathing a sigh of relief because their children are finally in college and stretching their wings, my 20 year-old is far from self-sufficient and may never be. Because she compensates so well, many people forget how challenged Kara is, or they assume she has grown out of the problems that surfaced in early childhood. When Kara was in twelfth grade it brought me to tears when excited and proud mothers would compare notes about the scholarships and college acceptance letters and ask me where my daughter was "going." Everyone, even those who were close to us, assumed she would have a scholarship to an art school. It broke my heart to acknowledge to them and to myself: another year of high school. That's where my kid was going. It was so hard for me to let go of the dream of college, and dorm life, and a career, but that was my dream, not Kara's.

So here we are. My beautiful, perfect daughter, my dream come true, is 20 years old. She has chosen to leave home, rather than follow the four house rules (don't lie, go to school and pass your classes, work, don't have your boyfriend over when I am not home). But she is safe. She is living with another family, in a nice neighborhood, and they support her emotionally and financially. She is not in jail, not using, not pregnant, and not on the streets. She finished high school and has nearly a year of community college credit. At age 20 the world is ready, whether or not I am, for Kara to make her own dreams come true.

CHAPTER 6

Child Welfare

FETAL ALCOHOL SPECTRUM DISORDERS, ADOLESCENTS, AND THE CHILD WELFARE SYSTEM

Sidney Gardner

Sidney Gardner, President of Children and Family Futures, Inc. and author of Beyond Collaboration to Results, offers an overview of the child welfare system in the U.S. and the impact of FASDs on the system. He explains in detail his realistic observation that, "Prenatal alcohol exposure can worsen the impact of foster care, and living in foster care can worsen the impact of prenatal alcohol exposure." He looks at children with FASDs in the foster care system and how together these issues relate to the school system, the mental health care system, adoptive parents, and the juvenile justice system.

INTRODUCTION

Of the 397,122 children in foster care as of September 30, 2012, a total of 127,061 (or 32%) were 13 to 18 years of age. An additional 6,036 were 19-20. These are the children who are:

- least likely to be adopted
- most likely to have lived in multiple placements
- most likely to have behavioral problems that affect their participation in school, combined with cognitive problems that affect their learning
- most likely to abuse drugs and alcohol
- most likely to have histories of trauma, often related to their parents' substance abuse and co-occurring domestic violence
- most likely to have children outside marriage.

Among these children, girls can be at added risk, due to sexual abuse, neglect of their physical and mental health, and various forms of trauma. Adolescents in the foster care system, like all children in that environment, have a higher risk of having been affected by prenatal exposure to alcohol and other drugs. A study of foster care children and youth in Washington State found that the rate of fetal alcohol syndrome was ten to fifteen times higher than in the general population.[1]

Foster and adoptive parents of these children often lack comprehensive histories of their children's genetic risks, trauma, or education. As a result, foster and adoptive parenting of these children presents many challenges for which these parents are not prepared, which can add to the risks that these children will not enter adulthood in stable families with the education and socio-emotional skills they need to succeed in life.

The other chapters in this collection have described the effects of Fetal Alcohol Spectrum Disorders (FASDs) on children and youth. For those who experience removal from their biological parents and placement in out-of-home care, the effects of the foster care system itself can compound those effects. Foster care involves further trauma for many children, not only in the dislocation of leaving their homes and their parents but in the challenges of meeting the demands made by the child welfare system on foster parents and agencies. Supervisory visits, review of health and educational services, periodic hearings to assess the prospects for reunification or termination of parental rights — all these necessary forms of oversight can affect children as new uncertainties and intrusions that add to the disruption of out-of-home care.

Prenatal alcohol exposure can worsen the impact of foster care, and living in foster care can worsen the impact of prenatal alcohol exposure. To the extent that rational decision-making and impulse control are weakened by the effects of alcohol exposure on the developing fetal brain, living in a controlled environment with rigid rules—the group home experience—can lead to rebellious behavior. And when foster care means an unstructured situation in a foster home with little supervision, in which caretakers or older relatives may have essentially given up, a youth with poor decision-making skills may have even less guidance on decisions about school, career, and relationships. Even when the child welfare system performs as it is intended to, achieving some measure of safety, permanency, and well-being, adolescents who have come through that system are compelled to cope with the next phases of their lives with numerous problems that may hamper their adjustment, lacking the ability:

> ...to think ahead to self-direct behavior, to maintain and integrate multiple bits of information, to stay on task, to problem

solve in an organized manner, or to place information in memory for later recall.[2]

SCREENING AND ASSESSMENT IN THE CHILD WELFARE SYSTEM
Federal and state law place a significant burden upon child welfare agencies to screen and assess the health and mental health needs of the children in foster care. Federal law requires states to certify that they have two separate types of screening processes for children in the child welfare system:
1. screening for prenatal exposure, including conditions that result from prenatal alcohol exposure, that affect newborns and younger children through two years of age, under the Child Abuse Prevention and Treatment Act (CAPTA) and;
2. referral for screening of all children under three with substantiated cases of abuse or neglect by the federally mandated agency responsible for younger children with developmental disabilities under the Individuals with Disabilities Education Act (IDEA).[3]

Yet there are very few states or localities that aggregate and report on the children who have been screened under these provisions, and the federal government itself does not monitor these totals across the states.

As described in earlier chapters, detection and diagnosis of FASDs is not a simple matter of a readily available test for a physical or mental disorder. Child welfare agencies respond to emergencies and reports of abuse or neglect, and clinical screening of the effects — or causes — of those emergencies and threats to safety are based on protocols and screening tools that rarely include detailed diagnostic assessments that would assess effects from prenatal alcohol exposure.

Nationally, detection of parental drug and alcohol use is highly variable, with one source finding that child welfare caseworkers missed 61% of all diagnosed substance use disorders.[4] States vary from those that do not report any parental substance abuse as a cause for removal of children to those that report more than half of their caseloads in this category. With overall substance use disorders among parents identified in such a variable pattern, recognition of the specific diagnoses that fall under the umbrella of FASDs is even more difficult.

Child welfare agencies are not public health organizations, nor do they typically possess ready access to pediatricians and other physicians or child psychiatrists familiar with FASDs. As noted in the literature on prenatal alcohol exposure, misdiagnosis of several other conditions can obscure the presence of FASDs in some children and youth. The "easier" diagnoses of attention deficit disorder, oppositional behavior, the autism spectrum, and bipolar disorders may take precedence, as the child welfare system relies on busy practitioners who may sometimes take months to actually see a referred child. Nor is it likely that the child welfare system will focus on the extent to which out-of-home care itself and the functioning of the child welfare system may contribute to some of these diagnoses. A recent review of out-of-home children in the child welfare system concluded that," It appears that child welfare system factors as well as biological factors significantly contribute to the occurrence of ADHD...."[5]

Schools, as discussed below, may have labeled children in a way that foster or adoptive parents seize upon as an explanation of what is "wrong" with their children, without probing for underlying causes such as prenatal exposure.

CHILD WELFARE SYSTEMS AND COORDINATION GAPS WITH OTHER AGENCIES

Child welfare is often at a disadvantage in being held accountable for results that can only be achieved with resources beyond its control. This is especially true since the child welfare system itself is only one of several agencies that have a role in diagnosing and treating FASDs—and it is arguably one of the less important ones. Many agencies and organizations other than child welfare have specific or potential responsibilities for identifying and intervening with potential or actual FASDs: maternal and child health, early childhood care and education, hospitals, health clinics, mental health practitioners, obstetricians, pediatricians and other children's health care providers, developmental disabilities, and schools. But very few of them, in the typical community or state, function as part of a well-connected network that recognizes its role in responding to FASDs among children and youth. As a result, the child welfare agency can be left without the resources or expertise these other agencies may have in recognizing and responding to FASDs.

These deficiencies in coordination and networking can be compounded by a tendency in child welfare agencies to adopt insular practices for what are very understandable reasons. Coordination with other agencies takes time, their resources are not easily made available for child welfare clients, and the difficulties of operating within the child welfare system are great enough without taking on the complexities of learning about other agencies' different mandates, eligibility criteria, funding streams, and political pressures.

As clear as it may seem to practitioners familiar with FASDs that no single agency can respond effectively to all the many aspects of an adolescent's life when that life is impacted by the effects of prenatal exposure to alcohol, a hard-pressed child welfare agency may view needed connections with other agencies as bridges too far to try to cross. For adolescents who may be close to leaving the system, there also may be a tendency among child welfare agencies to devote less attention to the other agencies and assume that they will pick up responsibility for these youth once they leave child welfare as a result of their age.

THE ROLE OF BIRTH, FOSTER AND ADOPTIVE PARENTS

Parents of adolescents with FASDs, whether birth, foster, or adoptive, may face problems distinguishing between "normal" adolescent resistance to authority and rebellious behavior and an inability to understand instructions or "follow the rules" due to alcohol's effects on the child's brain functioning. Adolescence is often a painful time for both youth and parents. The expected frustrations that come with the territory in the best of circumstances is only multiplied for parents of youth with FASDs as the parents deal on a daily basis with adolescents who won't comply with boundaries. Assuming that behavior is willful disobedience may confuse the effects of missed or misunderstood messages with rebellion, which may then lead to further demands and instructions, compounding the communication barriers.

Foster and adoptive parents of adolescents affected by their biological parents' substance abuse may exhibit a wide range of understanding of fetal alcohol effects, from those with very little awareness and understanding of the potential effects of prenatal exposure to those who are familiar with their children's history and the effects of that experience.[6] Child welfare agencies do not always share the full details of children in out-of-home placement when substance abuse is involved. At times, the agency is unaware of the details of the history of the children in their caseloads, even though their parents' substance abuse may be recorded in the case file. And some agencies deliberately withhold such information out of fears that foster and adoptive parents will conclude that such children are too difficult to parent. Few child welfare agencies refer parents to services that prepare parents to deal with the possible effects of prenatal exposure.

Foster and adoptive parents may struggle with understanding the effects of FASDs, and that struggle may worsen considerably as adolescents acquire new ways of being disruptive. A second-grader who is having difficulty learning and staying on task is very different from a high school junior who disrupts class, attends irregularly, disappears from the house with unapproved companions, and begins to encounter law enforcement and the juvenile justice system.

Nor should the critical role of biological parents be ignored in assessing the interaction between child welfare systems and adolescents affected by prenatal alcohol exposure. Since 85% of children with substantiated cases of abuse and neglect are either left at home or returned to their parents through reunification, these birth parents can be critical in helping their children adjust to adulthood, whether these parents achieve recovery or remain addicted.[7] Some of these returned children and youth then re-enter the child welfare system, worsening their sense of stability and their inability to see a life plan ahead.

Even when children are removed to permanency and parents' rights are terminated, older children without safe places to live may at times return to their birth parents once they have left the foster care system. This occurs both as young adults try to re-connect with undeniably important people in their lives and as they seek out a place to stay, even temporarily. The fact that one of the striking effects of prenatal alcohol exposure includes difficulties in processing new information in new settings makes returning home seem irrational in the long run. But these youth, in many ways, simply do not live in the long run. For those youth who have received preventive or rehabilitative treatment that has succeeded in turning them away from substance abuse, they may hold out hope that their biological parents are able to recover, too.

FOSTER CARE AND SCHOOL SYSTEMS' RESPONSES TO FASDs

A recurring issue affecting children in the foster care system is coordinating responses to their needs among parents, child welfare agencies, and school systems. The education of students in foster care typically yields results well below the norm. Considerable effort has been devoted recently to strengthening the ties between schools and child welfare agencies, including better information systems that track children across school systems when frequent moves may disrupt school attendance. Curricula have been developed that explain the effects of foster care to teachers and other school staff, underscoring the need for continuity in educational testing and class assignments as well as the risks of less parental supervision than other children may receive.[8-10] Yet materials focusing on the child welfare status of these children in school settings rarely mention prenatal exposure in any depth, with no discussion of alcohol effects. And materials on teaching students with FASDs rarely address the special circumstances of foster care status as it may complicate educational outcomes.

Special education status of students in foster care has been documented to be well above the average for all students. Special education students are reviewed periodically through an Individualized Education Plan (IEP) process that includes school staff, parents, and others involved in the care and education of the student. In the case of foster children, that can at times include the child welfare caseworker or another representative of the agency. But as noted, the special issues arising with alcohol-affected children and youth are typically not part of the special educational categories of need, which include several diagnostic categories that are designated by the school system as part of their compliance with the IDEA legislation and regulations. These categories do not include diagnoses within the fetal alcohol spectrum, and the overlaps between academic risk status due to prenatal alcohol exposure and the acceptable diagnoses of need are rarely reflected in an IEP. Thus the effects of FASDs on students with other diagnoses may be essentially invisible, obscured by placement in vague categories such as "other health impairment," which is a catch-all term used by some school districts for students who have disabilities that cannot be easily classified using current categories.

Foster and adoptive parents who lack concrete information about prenatal exposure or the issues of FASDs may be at a disadvantage in making the case for accommodations to the student's needs. For some parents the IEP process can be bewildering and intimidating, resulting in parents' becoming passive because they lack the leverage needed to deal with bureaucratic, time-consuming meetings and procedures. Those meetings are nearly always held during the workday, which adds to parents' inability to participate effectively. Some foster and adoptive parents have used educational advocates and/or attorneys with special education expertise to press their case for added services that the school district (and, in some states, the state or local mental health agency) may resist due to the added costs. When behavioral problems are involved, including those that may be a result of the young person's prenatal alcohol exposure, the school district may resort to suspension or expulsion as a way of ridding itself of the responsibility for the student.

Other problems faced by foster children in schools include difficulties in gaining credits when they have attended multiple schools or may have spent time in schools run by detention centers, group homes, or residential treatment centers. Getting prior transcripts sent to the current school is one set of challenges, and getting full credit for classes taken in a partial semester is another.[11] As students transition from one educational setting to another, the adolescent affected by FASDs may find it very difficult to navigate from one set of procedures, rules, and expectations to a new set, and may find it almost impossible to advocate for herself as these changes overwhelm her ability to process multiple sources of confusing information. Child welfare agencies, in turn, can be confused by educational processes developed in another service system with different goals and objectives, run by professionals from another discipline.

FOSTER CARE AND THE MENTAL HEALTH SYSTEM

Some foster and adoptive parents, either on their own or with guidance by the child welfare agency, may be able to connect their adolescent children with continuing mental health counseling. A result of this for many children in the child welfare system may be prescription of psychotropic drugs as part of a treatment plan. In some cases, stimulants may be prescribed for youth with attention deficit disorder, leading to calming effects for some, but affecting others in ways that may increase impulsive and erratic behavior. Hyperactive adolescents are not uniformly aided by stimulants, and the underground market for stimulants among college students and others is a reminder that these prescriptions can be abused in ways that the mental health practitioners do not intend.

In some states, the child welfare system and the mental health system have considerable difficulty getting on the same page about the appropriate treatment for a youth in out-of-home care. When special education status is involved, the confusion can multiply further, worsening the ability of the youth and his parents to understand the expectations and eligibility issues involved in working with the different systems. This confusion can overwhelm a youth with FASDs, making long-term planning for the future seem even more impossible when all these external actors exert controls.

FOSTER CARE AND THE JUVENILE DELINQUENCY SYSTEM

For "cross-over youth," the term used for those adolescents who are clients of the child welfare and the delinquency/juvenile justice systems at the same time, many of these issues are compounded. Impulsivity may have led to the youth with FASDs becoming involved with the juvenile justice system, and impulsivity may make it very difficult for that youth to imagine a future outside institutional life.

Like the child welfare system, diagnostic skills are not always present and available in the juvenile justice system. This can lead to labeling the youth as a trouble-maker, leading to tighter controls, which lead in turn to more impulsive reactions against incarceration or probation oversight. Child welfare systems may turn away from older youth in these situations, assuming that the youth is being cared for while incarcerated.

AGING OUT OF FOSTER CARE AND FASDs

Under the Fostering Connections Act of 2008, a Transition Plan for Emancipating Youth is to be developed during the 90-day period prior to a child's leaving the foster care system. Regulations require that the child's caseworker must develop a personalized transition plan that is "directed by the child." States have the option of keeping these youths' case plans open until they reach 21.

Independent living programs that prepare foster youth 15–17 years old for their departure from the foster care system are in force in most states. Some of these include information about substance abuse by the youth themselves, but very few address issues related to FASDs, and the literature on independent living programs devotes very little attention to this issue.[12,13] An otherwise excellent review of adolescent brain functioning reviewed the mental health issues and histories of trauma affecting many youth in foster care, referencing impact on the prefrontal cortex of the adolescent brain, without ever mentioning FASDs or prenatal exposure to alcohol or illicit drugs.[14]

Older youth and young adults with FASDs have further issues that arise when they are no longer subject to the legal systems governing minors. Sexual activity with minors, driven by impulsivity, can affect young adults who have been in the foster care system in which girls may have been abused in ways that make them especially vulnerable.

Even the best life skills preparation may not equip young adults or late teens with the tools they need to achieve stable employment, housing, higher education, and personal relationships. When the effects of FASDs are added to the effects of lengthy or often-interrupted stays in foster care, the prospects for independent living are diminished considerably for many of these young adults. Older youth in foster care have typically had more placements and thus more mobility and uncertainty in their lives.

Independence from foster care can mean relying on a low-paying job and living in low-cost housing in a troubled neighborhood without the educational tools or personal networks to improve the situation. In the short run, freedom from the restrictions of foster care and the oversight of the child welfare system may further impulsive and risky behavior, just as it does for many middle- and upper-income youth following graduation and leaving home and parental control to attend college. The lack of self-regulation skills among youth and young adults with FASDs can make these episodes of impulsive behavior more severe, running increased risks of substance abuse, unintended pregnancy, homelessness, or turning to criminal lifestyles.

Some excellent programs, modeled on the Guardian Scholars program first developed in the California state college system, have been able to gain access to two- and four-year colleges for some youth who have aged out of the foster care system.[15] But these programs have learned that continuing care and support are needed to cope with the problems created by a lack of study skills as well as living skills. Prenatal alcohol exposure can worsen those problems by adding the barrier of an inability to focus on lectures in college classrooms and homework assignments, planning a daily schedule, and preparing for tests and semester-long projects.

CONCLUSION

The challenges facing youth in the foster care system and those who have left that system can be considerably complicated by the effects of FASDs, in ways that the child welfare system often is not equipped to respond to effectively. Preparing reunified birth, foster, and adoptive parents to cope with issues related to FASDs is not a function that the child welfare system typically addresses in depth. The effects of foster care itself, combined with the effects of FASDs in older youth, can present many obstacles to these youth and those who seek to guide them to better lives. Yet models and best practices exist that can do a better job of diagnosing and responding to the dual effects of FASDs and foster care for adolescents. Child welfare systems and, of equal importance, the agencies they should be working with in serving older youth, need deeper awareness of the problems and development of strategies and opportunities to address the needs of adolescents affected by prenatal exposure to alcohol.

NOTES

1   Astley SJ, Stachowiak J, Clarren SK, Clausen C. Application of the fetal alcohol syndrome facial photographic screening tool in a foster care population. *Journal of Pediatrics,* 2002;141(5):712-7.

2   Chasnoff IJ, Wells AM, Telford E, Schmidt C, Messer G. Neurodevelopmental Functioning in Children With FAS, pFAS, and ARND *Journal of Developmental & Behavioral Pediatrics,* 2010;31(3):192-201.

3   http://www.acf.hhs.gov/cwpm/programs/cb/laws_policies/laws/cwpm/policy_dsp.jsp?citID=350

4   Gibbons CB, Barth RP, Martin SL. Substance abuse among caregivers of maltreated children. University of North Carolina at Chapel Hill; 2005. Unpublished manuscript .

5   Wells AM, Chasnoff IJ, Bailey GW, Jandasek B, Telford E, Schmidt C. Mental health disorders among foster and adopted children with FAS and ARND. Illinois Child Welfare Journal, in press, 2014.

6   The author and his wife have for the past twenty years been adoptive parents of two children from the child welfare system who are affected by their parents' substance use and their own prenatal exposure. Both children had special education diagnoses; one has been in several residential placements as well.

7   It should be noted that the rates of reunification of children prenatally exposed to alcohol or other drugs tend to be lower than these national averages.

8   Blaschke K, Maltaverne M, Struck J. "Fetal Alcohol Spectrum Disorders Education Strategies: Working with Students with a Fetal Alcohol Spectrum Disorder in the Education System." Center for Disabilities, Sanford School of Medicine of The University of South Dakota, 2009.

9   "A Resource Guide for Florida Educators Teaching Students with Fetal Alcohol Spectrum Disorders" Florida Department of Education Bureau of Exceptional Education and Student Services. 2005.

10 Leone P, Weinberg L. "Addressing the Unmet Educational Needs of Children and Youth in the Juvenile Justice and Child Welfare Systems" The Center for Juvenile Justice Reform, Georgetown University, 2010.

11 Leone and Weinberg, op.cit. 19.

12 The Mental Health of Vulnerable Youth and Their Transition to Adulthood: Examining the Role of the Child Welfare, Juvenile Justice, and Runaway/Homeless Systems, Child Trends, http://aspe.hhs.gov/hsp/09/YouthMentalHealth/Services/rb.pdf, 2009.

13 Hatton H, Brooks S. Factors, Characteristics, and Practices Related to Former Foster Youth and Independent Living Programs: A Literature Review. UC Davis Human Services Northern California Training Academy http://academy.extensiondlc.net/file.php/1/resources/LR-ILP.pdf, 2009.

14 The Adolescent Brain: New research and its implications for young people transitioning from foster care. Jim Casey Youth Opportunities Initiative, St. Louis, Mo., 2011.

15 http://www.orangewoodfoundation.org/programs_scholars.asp

CHAPTER 7

FASDs AND THE JUSTICE SYSTEM

Howard Davidson, J.D., and Katherine Kelly

Legal

Since more than half of those who live with FASDs find themselves, at some point in their lives, in trouble with the law, most for the first time as juveniles, learning why and how this happens is important for parents, caregivers, and professionals working with young people who have this disability.

> "We can envision few things more certainly beyond one's control than the drinking habits of a parent prior to one's birth"
>
> --Florida Supreme Court
> *Dillbeck v. State* (1994)
> 643 So.2d 1027, 1029

This chapter is excerpted, in part, from Chapter 7, FASD and the Law, by K.A. Kelly, from *Prenatal Alcohol Use and Fetal Alcohol Spectrum Disorders: Diagnosis, Assessment and New Directions in Research and Multimodal Treatment*, with permission from the publisher, and available from Bentham E-Books: http://benthamscience.com/ebooks/

GETTING IN TROUBLE WITH THE LAW: WHY AND HOW

In research conducted for the Centers for Disease Control and Prevention (CDC) by the University of Washington, Fetal Alcohol and Drug Unit, Dr. Ann Streissguth and colleagues found that approximately 60% of the 415 individuals studied, all of whom had been diagnosed with what was then known as fetal alcohol syndrome/fetal alcohol effects (FAS/FAE) and is now fetal alcohol spectrum disorders (FASDs), had been in trouble with the law.[1,2] For two-thirds of the individuals studied, an incident of law violation occurred first (or the only time) when they were under the age of 18. Another study[3] found that 23% of youth offenders, referred by Juvenile Court judges in British Columbia for a psychiatric/psychological assessment, had a prenatal alcohol-related diagnosis. They found 1% were diagnosed with FAS and 22.3% were diagnosed with what we would now term Fetal Alcohol Spectrum Disorders (FASDs). No young person was included in the study unless there was confirmation, by the mother or another reliable informant, of alcohol exposure in utero.

Most who parent or come to know someone well with FASDs have wondered why youth with FASDs so often "get in trouble with the law." The explanation, generally, can be found within the frequently observed behaviors that are typical of the disability; the young people are, very often, gullible, vulnerable, and young for their age. Their awkwardness in social settings makes it difficult for them to make and keep friends so they can be isolated and poignantly lonely. What better circumstance for exploitation by others could there be? So, heedless of consequences and eager to be accepted, the young person living with FASDs will follow the lead of non-disabled others into criminal activity and will be apprehended for violating the law when the others, sensing danger, have fled.

Or, in other situations, because impulse control can be a problem for them, they will see some attractive item and may unlawfully appropriate it, never considering what penalties may lie in store for them. Couple such impulsivity with frequent frustration, leading to explosive anger, and one can see the possibility of incidents of assault against another person, generally someone smaller in size. Bullied when younger, they can become bullies as they age and grow. And, because those with FASDs have undependable, impaired memories and difficulty learning from their mistakes, they may repeat, again and again, the same foolish and hurtful behaviors.

Youth with FASDs are frequently apprehended when they are found to be shoplifting, often ineptly. They are very likely to be noticed when they offend, since they can be noisy, talkative, physically awkward, and inappropriate. They are usually not good at stealth or in exercising discretion. And, generally, they cannot plan a multi-step offense, so if they are involved in such, more competent peers likely have brought them into it. Often, if a group has been apprehended, the non-disabled perpetrators will identify the disabled individual as the leader, will plead guilty, and will agree to testify against the disabled youth in exchange for a reduced penalty. The individual with FASDs will then tend to take the blame for his or her associates, perhaps in hopes that this will promote good will and gratitude from the individuals they consider to be their "friends."

The most serious offenses, in their consequences to both the victims and to the offenders with FASDs, are sexual offenses. Research[1,2] has shown that for those ages 12–20, about 40% of both young men and young women with FAS become involved in inappropriate sexual behavior, while about 50% of young men and 55% of young women within the overall fetal alcohol spectrum have been involved in inappropriate sexual behavior. Of those females who exhibited inappropriate sexual behaviors, the prevalence of sexual victimization among them was between 80% and 90%. For males, the victimization rate was 50% to 60%. Victims themselves as children, those with FASDs may, as they grow older, become involved in the victimization of others.[3]

Sex offenses committed by those with FASDs often occur, in part, because of significant immaturity and very poor judgment. A young man may, for example, become involved in a "consensual" sexual relationship with a young woman who is very much below the age of consent. It is alarming that these young offenders, who may be chronologically age 17, but age 9 or 10 developmentally, may serve lengthy terms as sexual predators in juvenile correctional facilities, or worse, in adult prisons; and then they will be required to register as sex offenders, with all that implies.

Youth with FASDs also may become involved in the juvenile justice system due to their experimentation with or addiction to unlawful substances, as well as offenses related to excessive alcohol consumption. Research[4] with rat pups exposed prenatally to ethanol showed that if the exposed adolescent rats were offered a variety of beverages, including ethanol, they would seek out the ethanol. It was demonstrated that the exposed animal's avidity to ethanol was directly attributable to an altered perception of ethanol's normally aversive odor and bitter-like flavor. Ethanol's odor and taste were familiar to the animals from ingesting it and absorbing it during their gestation. However, if the animals were not offered ethanol in their adolescence and were only offered it once they reached adulthood, the preference for ethanol had been suppressed and the rats did not seek it out. The suggestion, then, is that if human adolescents with FASDs do not use alcohol in their teens, they will not have an increased susceptibility to alcohol and vulnerability to alcohol addiction in adulthood.

Among 12–20 year-olds with FAS, over 30% of males and 5% of females have either alcohol or other drug problems.[1,2] Of those in this age group with other diagnoses within FASDs, 30% of males and slightly less than 40% of females have alcohol and other drug problems. When those with FASDs enter a typical program for addiction treatment, their disability can make sobriety a frustrating quest.[5] The disabled youth's lack of focus, difficulty following interactions in a group, sometimes slow processing speed, lack of introspection, impaired reading and written expression, and impulsivity, coupled with the addiction professionals' typical lack of awareness regarding FASDs, often make these youth "program failures." Is the disabled individual failing the program, or is the program failing the disabled individual?

A youth with FASDs also may come into contact with the juvenile justice system by purportedly being beyond the control of a parent or caregiver,[6,7] e.g., slipping out of the house repeatedly at night, running away, chronic truancy, having tantrums escalating into rages or physical aggression toward a younger sibling or parent. Parents seeking help from the court for their child's out-of-control behavior can seem to them a logical step, especially when other options have been exhausted. It is, however, very important that courts hearing a "status offender" petition based on the misbehavior at home of a youth with suspected FASDs order appropriate assessments to identify a young person's areas of strength and areas of deficit, in order to develop an individualized and effective intervention program.

JUVENILE COURT

Turning to the courts for help with their out-of-control child, or finding that their child with FASDs has committed a criminal offense, may be quite traumatic for a parent or caregiver, but it also can be an opportunity. This may be the first time a young person with FASDs has come into contact with a government agency with a mission that includes, among other goals, helping the young person obtain needed services and assistance.

Officials in the juvenile justice system may be uniquely able to arrange for services and assistance from federal, state, and local agencies.[8] Parents, caregivers, and professionals working with a youth with FASDs should encourage juvenile justice and court officials to help in this way, stressing that they may have access and leverage that the parents do not. Lawyers representing young people with FASDs should act as effective advocates, arguing that getting relevant assistance will advance the court's interest in preventing recidivism. The observed respect that most individuals with FASDs have for authority figures can be turned to a good purpose. A youth with FASDs might be particularly responsive to admonitions and supervision by a judge, who may be able to guide the defendant's actions—and encourage him or her—in a way that parents or others cannot.

On the other hand, the consequences of getting in trouble with the law can be extremely destructive. Individuals with FASDs are particularly vulnerable to victimization while detained, with psychological consequences that may significantly impair their future behavior.[3] They simply cannot discern what socially appropriate behavior is, and they may be very irritating to their fellow residents. This can result in the disabled youth becoming the victim of assaults while detained. Corrections staff may then, for the youth's protection, place her or him in segregation, causing even more psychological harm. Thus, youth with FASDs who are detained for lengthy periods may be, upon release, more impaired and dysfunctional than they were when initially institutionalized.

There is enormous variation in the degree to which lawyers, prosecutors, judges, probation officers and other court professionals know about FASDs, or understand how it might have affected the conduct of a youth or how it could impact his future behavior. Obtaining the most appropriate treatment of a defendant with FASDs—and avoiding recidivism—may depend, to a significant degree, on the ability of an advocate (e.g., a lawyer dealing with a judge, or a parent talking to a police officer, lawyer or probation officer) to offer a convincing explanation of FASDs and its connection to a child's juvenile justice system involvement.[9-12]

Encouraging FASDs awareness, the American Bar Association in

2012 approved a policy resolution[13] urging "attorneys and judges, state, local, and specialty bar associations, and law school clinical programs to help identify and respond effectively to Fetal Alcohol Spectrum Disorders in children and adults, through training to enhance awareness of FASDs and its impact on individuals in the child welfare, juvenile justice, and adult criminal justice systems and the value of collaboration with medical, mental health, and disability experts." It also urged the passage of laws and adoption of policies at all levels of government that acknowledge and treat the effects of prenatal alcohol exposure and better assist individuals with FASDs.[13] The U.S. Department of Health and Human Services has supported publication of several materials addressing these issues and the best ways of helping juvenile defendants with FASDs.[14]

LEGAL ISSUES
Culpability Under the Law

The Canadian Bar Association has pointed out that "[T]he criminal justice system is based on normative assumptions that a person acts in a voluntary manner, makes informed choices with respect to the decision to commit crimes, and learns from their own behavior and the behavior of others…[T]hese normative assumptions and the sentencing principles such as specific and general deterrence are not valid for those with FASDs…."[15]

Whether FASDs may support a defense of diminished capacity depends on the state law standard for that defense, and on the nature of the underlying offense.[16] Individuals with FASDs are impulsive, and have difficulty thinking ahead to plan and organize their activities. The existence of this disability could be highly relevant to whether a juvenile had premeditated an act, or was actually innocent of an act that would have required significant planning and preparation. In most cases, these issues are not litigated at trial. Rather, the attorney for the youth may rely on this type of information and legal reasoning to negotiate a more humane and effective case settlement and dispositional plan.[17,18]

False Confessions

Individuals with FASDs, because of their disability, are more likely to confess to crimes that they did not commit, or crimes which did not even occur. There are several reported court decisions in which this occurred, and more cases which are unreported.[19] This problem occurs in part because individuals with FASDs are very suggestible as well as extremely anxious to please interrogators or other authority figures. They may confuse events that actually occurred with stories recounted to them by the police or others.

Even when an individual with FASDs understands that the confession he or she is being asked to sign is not correct, he may do so with the naïve misunderstanding, perhaps fostered by the police, that there will be no consequences to the confession. Those two problems are interconnected; a non-disabled person who wanted to please a police officer, but was mindful of the consequences, might be exceptionally polite to a police officer, but would not confess to a crime that he did not commit. Similarly, a person who did not have FASDs would not believe a police officer's assurance that he could just go home without any further consequences after confessing to a serious crime.

The false confession situation is illustrated with painful clarity by the prosecution of Gabriel B., who was diagnosed as a teenager with FAS.[20] Mr. B, then 18, pled guilty to, and was convicted of, a serious arson at the high school he was attending (in Special Education) in Washington State. A state psychiatric hospital subsequently examined him and concluded, in part because he seemed unwilling to acknowledge his culpability, that he was a threat to the community. Two years after Mr. B.'s conviction, another individual came forward and confessed to the crime, exhibiting knowledge of events that only the arsonist could have had. Mr. B. was exonerated; prosecutors admitted that they had made a mistake, dropped the charges, and asked the court to overturn his conviction.

The transcript of the police interrogation makes crystal clear that, when asked about the offense, Mr. B. was entirely unable to describe the manner or location in which the fire had been started; only when the police repeatedly corrected his mistaken descriptions did Mr. B. finally give the correct answers. The police officers seemed to have been oblivious to the fact that—in a taped interview—they were feeding the answers to the suspect. The officers seemed more motivated by a desire to be helpful to a perpetrator they perceived as having a poor memory than to obtain a confession from him at all costs. Mr. B. later explained that he knew at the time that he had not started the fire, but told the police what they wanted to hear so he could go home as he had been promised.

Competence to Stand Trial
The competency of a defendant with FASDs to stand trial, and to assist with his or her own defense, is not simply a matter of IQ. Individuals with FASD generally function at a level below that typical of others with the same IQ. A recent U.S. Supreme Court decision in Hall v. Florida holds that an IQ score is not a determination of the intellectual capacity of the individual.[21] This is especially relevant since the adaptive behavior (how they function) of those with FASDs may be significantly more compromised than their IQ score would suggest. Competency to stand trial requires that the defendant have the capacity to understand the nature and object of the proceedings against her or him and to consult with counsel and assist in preparing his defense. Additionally, the defendant must have a sufficient present ability to consult with her or his lawyer with a reasonable degree of rational understanding and a rational as well as factual understanding of the proceedings against her or him. Due process requires a judge to hold a competency hearing whenever the evidence before the court raises a reasonable doubt as to whether a defendant is mentally competent.

An understanding of this issue should therefore focus not merely on general competency, but on three problems likely to affect a juvenile defendant with FASDs.[16-18,22] First, does the defendant have a clear enough grasp of the distinction between reality and fiction to be able to direct counsel in her or his defense and assist counsel in evaluating and responding to testimony or argument about what occurred? Second, does the defendant have a sufficient grasp of cause and effect so that he or she understands the effect of actions that he or she wants the attorney to take? Third, does the defendant understand what is taking place in the courtroom? For a juvenile defendant with FASDs to understand what is transpiring during the hearing and its implications, the court may need to take regular recesses to allow for "interpretive" assistance to be provided to the youth. An effective "interpreter" might be a Special Education teacher or other expert who has been trained in communicating with the cognitively disabled.

The role of the attorney for a juvenile in a delinquency proceeding is to advocate for the client's expressed preferences, not what is perceived to be in their best interests. When the competency of the youth to make decisions in her or his own best interest is in serious question, the court has the authority to appoint a *Guardian Ad Litem* (GAL) to advocate for the client's best interest. If it decides that the facts clearly warrant appointment of a GAL because of the child's incompetency, the court should make every effort to appoint a GAL who is knowledgeable about FASDs and how the disability may manifest itself in the young person's thinking processes.

Attorneys may request that the court order (and pay for) a diagnostic assessment regarding FASDs if there has not already been such an assessment. The court can also order, at the request of the attorney, a psychiatric/psychological evaluation if there is a question of the competency of the young person to stand trial, to determine if there is a basis for a diminished capacity or insanity defense, to determine if the youth had the capacity to waive the required *Miranda* warnings, or if the mental state of the youth might be a mitigating condition at sentencing.

Sentencing Dispositions

The relevance of a diagnosis of FASDs to juvenile sentencing, and to developing an effective sentencing plan, depends at the outset on the nature and elements of juvenile sentencing statutes. As a practical matter, FASDs might be very relevant to sentencing for the following reasons:[14-18,22,23]

(a) Individuals with FASDs may be less culpable under state standards. They may not fully understand the relevant norms of conduct; ignorance of the law may not be a defense, but an incomplete ability to understand the standards of conduct bears on culpability. Some offenses by individuals with

FASDs may be the result of impulsive behavior, over which the offender had less control than non-disabled defendants.

(b) The existence of FASDs may be important in determining what role a defendant played in an offense. Sophisticated criminals can talk individuals with FASDs into taking part in offenses they may not understand. The young person with FASDs may also, when questioned by investigators, accept responsibility for performing a more active role in the offense than actually occurred. She may believe her "friends" will be grateful or that she has hidden her disability from the questioner.

(c) The existence of FASDs may be critical in designing a sentence or sentencing alternative that will reduce the risk of recidivism and will avoid causing far greater harm to a defendant with FASDs than would be inflicted on a non-disabled defendant. Sentencing a youth with FASDs to a correctional facility will not teach the young person a lesson likely to deter future offenses if the individual does not fully understand why he or she has been incarcerated.

The Canadian Bar Association has observed that traditional "sentencing options available to courts are often ineffective in changing the behavior of those with FASDs..." and that incarceration may serve "...no rehabilitative or deterrent purpose.... [T]hose with FASDs [are] judged on a standard that they are incapable of meeting because of their disability."[15]

Transfer of Juveniles to Adult Court
Transferring a young person with FASDs who is under the age of 18 from juvenile to adult criminal court can be destructive and counterproductive, even where the offense is serious. Subsequent commitment to an adult jail or prison presents a particularly great danger to those with FASDs since imprisonment places a highly credulous individual with a disability into close and repeated contact with more sophisticated offenders. The individual with FASDs may come to regard these fellow inmates as his friends and may be lured into criminal schemes through this supposed friendship. In this respect, placing an individual with FASDs, whose maturity level may be

12 or 13, in a jail or prison is like imprisoning a child of that age, something that the law absolutely forbids and that, hopefully, no sensible judge would ever consider. One possible way to argue against such incarceration would be to arrange for a full battery of testing to assess the level of maturity of a defendant and, then, point to state laws setting the minimum age of persons who can be held with the adult population in a penal facility.

Individuals with FASDs are extremely impressionable. They are prone to modeling themselves on those with whom they have contact and to replicating behavior—including criminal behavior—that they see, hear about, or experience. Because of their impairments, individuals with FASDs are very vulnerable to physical and sexual abuse in prison, resulting in harms that could translate into further behavioral deterioration upon release. Placing an individual with FASDs in an institution in which many of the contacts will be with adult offenders (or even simply with serious juvenile offenders) runs a substantial risk that the individual will pose a greater danger to society after incarceration than before. That danger is all the greater if the individual develops relationships with fellow inmates who continue the pattern of law violation when returned to the community and with whom he might be in contact after release.

HOW TO WORK WITH JUVENILE COURT PROFESSIONALS

Unlike the adult criminal justice system, the juvenile justice system is generally focused on steps to prevent future offenses and to rehabilitate a juvenile offender, rather than inflicting punishment as retribution and for protection of the public. Juvenile court officials are generally more willing to respond to suggestions from parents and family members about the steps that should be taken in dealing with a juvenile offender. If a child with FASDs becomes involved with the juvenile justice system, parents should be aggressive in identifying programs and services the child needs—including programs and services that will continue into adulthood. They should advocate for help in establishing their child's eligibility for those programs and services.

The methods that will be effective in preventing recidivism by children with FASDs often will be significantly different than the approaches that would work best for children who do not have this disability. Judges, attorneys and probation officers should be alerted to the nature of this disability and urged to consider modifications of the usual approaches in order to be effective with those diagnosed with FASDs. Juvenile probation officers in particular need to be trained to recognize, and respond appropriately to, FASDs.

Two programs operating in juvenile courts in Minnesota and Colorado screened all youth referred to probation for FASDs. Those with a positive screen and confirmation of alcohol exposure in utero were referred to a multi-disciplinary FASDs diagnostic team for assessment. If the young person met criteria for diagnosis within FASDs, the youth was given a modified supervision plan that included closer oversight, more prompts to assist the probationer in successfully completing probation requirements, and an extension of probation for any new offense (rather than sanctions for probation violations, which as discussed below can be counterproductive for youth with FASDs). There was an understanding that the youth was disabled and not making conscious choices of noncompliance. Although this could run counter to defense attorneys' customary arguments for the least restrictive sentence possible, both the court and the attorneys were persuaded by the literature on FASDs demonstrating the value of lengthy, close and compassionate supervision. A review of the programs found, one to three years after the successful completion of such modified probation, the recidivism rate of those who had been given modified probation, was 15% versus the typical 50% recidivism rate for the court.

Individuals with FASDs often fare poorly on probation if the supervising officer does not understand their disability and fails to take it into account.[24] Probationers with FASDs generally have great difficulty keeping their appointments with their probation officers or with others such as drug testing agencies. The problem stems not from an unwillingness to meet these obligations, but rather from a significant incapacity to remember these obligations or to manage time in a way that permits the individual to appear as directed. Punishing these youth for their inability to keep their appointments; to appear on time; to submit monthly reports; to fulfill court orders; to attend school regularly or perform community service; to find and maintain work; to pay a fine; restitution, or court fees is generally pointless. Fear of punishment will not eliminate the disability that prevents an individual from complying.

The more appropriate and effective method for dealing with this problem is for the probation officer or others to offer strong and practical support to aid the disabled young person in meeting the obligations imposed on him by the court order. Examples include providing reminders by telephone, text messages, and emails to the individual of what he is supposed to do and when. Written lists that a probationer can post on the refrigerator with probation conditions written in positive, plain-English terms can be helpful. Judge Michael Jeffery, presiding over the Superior Court in Barrow, Alaska, has simplified his court documents, including his probation orders. Samples can be provided to the court, the attorney, and the probation officer for a youth with FASDs.[11]

A probation plan for a young Seattle man diagnosed with FASDs as a child and living with his grandmother included a daily, brief check-in with his probation officer followed by a GED class conducted by the probation department together with frequent drug testing. This young man very slowly worked toward his goal of receiving his GED, provided clean drug tests, and developed a close relationship with his probation officer and the other officers and staff. He did not re-offend and his probation supervision was closed. He still occasionally will stop by the office for a visit.

Since individuals with FASDs generally benefit from a closer and possibly a more prolonged period of supervision, whether on probation or after custodial release, than might ordinarily be provided to or warranted for other juvenile offenders, cautious, diligent and, perhaps, skeptical attorneys need to be provided with information explaining FASDs and why there is a need for structure, oversight, monitoring, and support if the best possible outcome for their client is to be achieved. Individuals with FASDs have, for example, expressed their reliance on drug testing, using the requirement to explain to their peers why they cannot use any proscribed substances. In serious cases in which detention might be likely, electronic monitoring, if available as an alternative, can be a highly useful component of supervision for a person with FASDs. Appointment reminders, explicit directions, concrete language, repetition of expected behaviors and non-punitive flexibility in responding to failure to fulfill probation obligations can all yield greater supervision success for a youth with FASDs.

As discussed earlier, one important factor that should also be considered in dealing with juvenile offenders is that youth with FASDs have great difficulty making appropriate friends, since they often lack key social skills. Cut off from developing friendships with most of their peers, adolescents with FASDs may by default associate with other juveniles with behavioral problems. Or, more sophisticated, non-disabled peers may "befriend" them in an effort to exploit them. Individuals with this disability do not have the social skills to discern when they are being "used" and can be drawn into new law violations in a futile attempt to follow the directions of their "friends." An approach[25] to assist these young people in developing relationships with pro-social peers and to avoid recidivism involves identifying a peer advocate or mentor (either volunteer or paid) who can provide companionship for a juvenile with FASDs. Possible sources for these mentors include churches, volunteer groups, high school counselors who can identify potential student volunteers, and college student employment offices where students majoring in psychology might be found. These volunteers also can provide tutoring and educational support.

"Contingency management" techniques may be effective tools to induce juveniles with FASDs who have been in trouble with the law to act in a more constructive manner.[26] Contingency management provides small material incentives for good behavior such as clean drug tests or regular school attendance. Gift cards for coffeehouses, bookstores, department stores, grocery stores have all been utilized in drug treatment programs and in court. These techniques have proven to be highly effective and could be used to reinforce compliance with probation requirements.

WORKING WITH THE CHILD'S ATTORNEY

One of the recurring problems that arises when an individual with FASDs gets in trouble with the law is the often difficult relationship between the individual's parents and his attorney. Unless an effective, cooperative relationship can be established, there is a greatly reduced likelihood that the juvenile justice system will deal appropriately with the defendant.

Attorneys for juvenile defendants are the key means of presenting information and arguments to the juvenile justice system, of identifying or developing the kind of information the system cares about, and putting it in a form that will be effective. Most attorneys, however, do not know anything about FASDs: what it is, how to detect it, or why it might be relevant to a juvenile case.[11,24]

In practice, only family members or close family friends usually are aware that a youth has FASDs, are able to see a connection between FASDs and the alleged proscribed conduct, and can articulate the likely consequences of possible sentences (or plea agreements) for the young person. The attorney representing a child with FASDs will need information and advice from the client's parents or other family members, and those family members often will be more than willing to provide that assistance.

Most attorneys, however, are wary, in part due to ethical concerns, of taking advice about legal tactics from a juvenile's family members. Time and again, defense attorneys have had to fend off ill-considered advice or misinformation from a client's family. The parents of even guilty clients routinely tell the attorney that their child is innocent or, at the least, misunderstood. This may be the case for someone with FASDs, but defense attorneys instinctively shun such advice and assistance. It is not unusual for the parents of a child with FASDs, acting in what they perceive to be the best interests of their child, to so annoy their child's attorney that the lawyer either withdraws from the case or refuses to talk further with the parents. The challenge then is for family members or other advocates to find a way to overcome this barrier to helping the young person's attorney understand the relevance of prenatal alcohol exposure.

Parents and guardians can take several steps to enhance the likelihood of a constructive relationship with the attorney representing their child. First, parents should collect relevant documents in order to provide the attorney with confirmation of the child's life-long disability. The lawyer will be more persuaded by documents revealing an atypical history than by pleading phone calls from a parent. The lawyer, moreover, needs documents to persuade a prosecutor to accept a more favorable disposition, plea agreement, or constructive sentence; the lawyer cannot rely on stories or explanations that she has simply heard from the client's parents.

The key documents to provide to the attorney include: (a) an FASDs diagnostic report, (b) special education or other illuminating school records, (c) social services agency or medical records indicating that the defendant has some type of cognitive problem, and (d) birth records indicating that alcohol was present at the time of the child's birth or that the baby was impaired in some way. Also include materials that explain what parents and advocates can do when a child with FASDs faces the juvenile court system. Copies of these materials should be provided to the lawyer in a notebook or folder, with the originals retained.

Second, it is important to recognize that the lawyer, by training and ethical responsibility, will not want family members and friends deciding legal tactics. The family should provide all relevant documents or other information to the attorney, and make clear to the attorney that the parents are willing to work cooperatively with probation officials and the court to support a supervision plan designed for their child with FASDs. Parents can be critical partners with the court and probation (after all, they know the child best) in developing and implementing a creative, flexible, tailored, effective supervision plan.

WHEN A JUVENILE WITH FASDs BECOMES A VICTIM

The disabilities of individuals with FASDs, both as children and as adults, render them easy prey for criminal conduct.[3] They are likely to accept criminal abuse, or to refrain from complaining to authorities, because they do not fully understand the inappropriateness of their mistreatment, or because they want to avoid displeasing the offender. A child with FASDs might fail to grasp the importance of parental admonitions against sexual contacts with adults, and to recognize a high level of danger in a situation. Some

72% of adolescents and adults with FASDs have been physically or sexually abused.[1,2]

Prosecuting an offender for victimizing an individual with FASDs may be complicated by difficulties preparing and relying on testimony from the victim. As witnesses, as in other aspects of their lives, individuals with FASDs are both credulous and very eager to please. A victim-witness with FASDs may believe that the correct response to a question must be whatever answer the questioner may appear to want, whether or not the response is factually true. Thus police and prosecutors must exercise great care in interviewing these young victims, taking pains not to lead them in any particular direction but, rather, inducing them to tell their own stories.

HELP FOR THOSE YOUTH LIVING WITH FASDs

Congress has established a national Protection and Advocacy (P&A) System to aid individuals with disabilities throughout their lifespan and in all aspects of their lives. There are 57 federally mandated P&A offices in the U.S., including states, U.S. Trust Territories and Associated States that offer advice and assistance on a wide range of issues, including special education, community living, financial entitlements, health care, sheltered and other employment and residential facilities. P&A offices serve those with FASDs and can assist those living with FASDs to access the help they need related to community integration (access to housing), criminal and juvenile justice system involvement (diversion, appropriate placement, conditions of confinement, and access to appropriate re-entry services), education, accommodations in general education and extracurricular activities, access to services required by the Individuals with Disabilities Education Act, and many other issues.

Assistance in obtaining vocational rehabilitation is provided under a related system of national offices, the Client Assistance Program (CAP). CAP and P&A agencies often are located in the same facility. Lawyers in P&A and CAP agencies can provide (without charge) legal help and other advocacy services to people with disabilities. They do not, however, represent clients in adult criminal or juvenile court proceedings. There have been instances when just a simple telephone call to a school from a P&A attorney could persuade school officials to move forward on a stalled request for an Individualized Education Plan. Information about the location and telephone number for the P&A and CAP office in each state can be obtained at the Website for the National Disability Rights Network, an organization of these agencies.[27] That website also explains in greater detail the work of the agencies and other programs for individuals with disabilities.

WHEN PARENTAL CARE AND CUSTODY ARE AFFECTED BY HAVING A CHILD WITH FASDs
Loss of Parental Rights

Most if not all states have statutes under which authorities can institute an action to terminate the rights of parents who are unable to safely care for their children. The standards under which a court can terminate parental rights vary. If the court terminates parental rights, the child is then typically legally freed for adoption. In proceedings to terminate parental rights, FASDs may be relevant in either or both of two ways. First, if the parent or parents themselves have FASDs, the court may regard that as some evidence of—or an explanation of—their inability to safely care for their child. Second, if the child in question has FASDs, the court may regard that as demonstrating that the child has special needs which require a heightened level of parenting skills. State court decisions regarding these problems are one of the largest categories of judicial opinions dealing with FASDs.

There is, however, no distinct legal issue applicable in this context to parents or children with FASDs. Rather, a disability due to prenatal alcohol exposure is simply a factual circumstance which may affect the abilities of the parent or parents, or the level of needs of the child. FASDs thus represent the source of certain types of practical problems. Those problems often have significant and effective practical solutions.

There are a number of programs, and a substantial body of experience, which courts and attorneys should look to in dealing with children with FASDs.[28] These children can be more challenging to raise; they have special needs, and the best ways of coping with those needs are often far from obvious. Parents of children with FASDs should not forfeit their parental rights simply because they cannot personally devise on their own all the creative approaches and strategies that clinicians and other parents have developed.

Similarly, although some parents with FASDs may experience difficulty raising a non-disabled child, there is also a body of experience regarding how to assist and guide those parents in caring for their children. The Parent-Child Assistance Program (P-CAP), which began in Washington State and has been replicated in a number of other states and many sites in Canada, provides assistance to these parents with disabilities.[10,28]

Guardianship After the Child Turns 18

In some states it is possible for a parent or a state agency (such as the state developmental disability agency) to be named guardian of an adult child with FASDs. Whether that is the right thing for a parent to do, or even attempt to do, is a difficult question. Depending on state law, a guardian might be able to make medical decisions, manage funds, or have the right to be involved in decision-making in a criminal proceeding. On the other hand, being placed under the supervision of a guardian could offend or demoralize some individuals. Parents and family members often are concerned as to a guardian's liability for the actions of the individual with FASDs; whether and when that might be the case would vary with state law. In assessing the right choice, the degree to which the individual with FASDs is disabled would undoubtedly be a major consideration. The laws on guardianship vary from state to state.

Recently, Illinois state law was modified to add FASDs to the list of the conditions that would warrant creating a guardianship.[30] That statute expanded the definition of "disabled person," for whom guardianship can be ordered, to include a person who "is diagnosed with fetal alcohol syndrome or fetal alcohol effects."

FINAL THOUGHTS

Because there is no research on what interventions for adolescents living with FASDs are most effective to prevent or ameliorate the effects of trouble with the law, these thoughts come from practice-based evidence rather than evidence-based practice. It seems, from observing the development of children with FASDs, that the maturation process simply takes a decade (or more) longer than the process for children without this disability. Think of the need to protect children with FASDs from harm beginning at birth and continuing to age 30, rather than the birth to 18 or 21 age range that we think of for those unaffected by prenatal alcohol exposure. There may be a physical explanation for this, as explained in previous chapters in this book, and it may be that the injured brain, as with a stroke victim, needs time to re-wire itself and find new pathways for functioning.

Whatever is taking place, parents, caregivers, and professionals working with youth with FASDs may not anticipate a developmental trajectory that includes practical emancipation at 18 or even 21. A warm, supportive family that expects the period of adolescence to last until age 30 may offer the greatest protection from trouble with the law. The idea that a disabled young person should be given increased freedom and encouraged to be fully independent may not be a workable strategy for those with FASDs, no matter how often the parent is characterized as over-protective or (in a pejorative way) accused of enabling. As in everything about those with FASDs, strategies around responding to law violations need to be different. A schedule for supervised activity 24/7 including school, personal interests, sports, a peer mentor, tutoring, and even sheltered or supported employment may offer a way forward that can protect the disabled young person from their poor decision-making, impaired judgment and insufficiently developed social skills.

Even if problems arise and a youth does get in trouble with the law, a community-based solution (probation, electronic monitoring in more severe cases to lieu of incarceration, addiction treatment) rather than detention, placement in a correctional facility, or transfer from juvenile to adult court, seem to be the very best hope for a favorable outcome. If the juvenile court can be helped to recognize that the best way to keep these young people from becoming chronic offenders is to keep them closely supervised in the community, the prospects for many youth with FASDs may be much improved. Family, caregiver and societal acceptance of an extended adolescence for the individual living with FASDs may well give the young person a chance, over time, to see what he has to work with as he goes about developing a productive life. This approach is supported by the experience of many families who are devoting their talent, energies, resources and love to navigating uncharted waters on behalf of these vulnerable youth.

NOTES

1	Streissguth AP, Barr HM, Kogan JK, Bookstein FL. Secondary disabilities in people with FAS and FAE. In: Streissguth AP, Kanter J, editors. The Challenge of Fetal Alcohol Syndrome: Overcoming Secondary Disabilities. Seattle: University of Washington; 1997

2	Streissguth AP, Barr H, Kogan J, Bookstein FL. Understanding the Occurrence of Secondary Disabilities in Clients with Fetal Alcohol Syndrome (FAS) and Fetal Alcohol Effects (FAE). Final Report to the Centers for Disease Control and Prevention. Grant #R04/CCR008515. Seattle: University of Washington School of Medicine; 1996.

3	Conry JL, Fast DK, Loock CA. Youth in the criminal justice; identifying FAS and other developmental disabilities. Vancouver BC: Final Report to the Ministry of the Attorney General; 1997.

4	Youngentob S. Fetal ethanol exposure increases ethanol intake by making it smell and taste better *Proc Natl Acad Sci U.S.A.* 2009:106, 5359-5364.

5	U.S. Department of Health and Human Services, Substance Abuse and Health Services Administration, Center for Substance Abuse Prevention. Fetal Alcohol Spectrum Disorders: curriculum for addiction professionals: Level 2, facilitators manual; 2007.

6	Streissguth AP. *Fetal Alcohol Syndrome: A guide for families and communities.* Baltimore: Paul H. Brookes Publishing Company; 1997

7	LaDue R, Dunne T. Legal issues and the Fetal Alcohol Syndrome. The FEN Pen Fall 1995; 6-7.

8	Fast DK, Conry JL. Fetal Alcohol Spectrum Disorders and the criminal justice system. *Developmental Disabilities Research Reviews* 2009;15:250-257.

9	Dubovsky D, McDonell M. FASD and Addition Treatment: Improving Outcomes. http://ihs.adobeconnect.com/p7c4p1sm8wy/.

10	Fetal Alcohol Unit of the University of Washington: http://depts.washington.edu/fadu

11	American Bar Association Center on Children and the Law at: http://www.americanbar.org/groups/child_law/what_we_do/projects/child_and_adolescent_health/fasd.html.

12 FASD Ontario Justice Committee: http://fasdjustice.ca/.

13 American Bar Association. http://www.americanbar.org/groups/child_law/tools_to_use/ attorneys/fasd-resolution.html.

14 Substance Abuse and Mental Health Services Administration. *Fetal Alcohol Spectrum Disorders and Juvenile Justice: How Professionals Can Make A Difference, Fetal Alcohol Spectrum Disorders: When Your Child Faces the Juvenile Justice System, Fetal Alcohol Spectrum Disorders and The Criminal Justice System:* http://fasdcenter.samhsa.gov/grabGo/factSheets.aspx.

15 Canadian Bar Association, Resolution 10-02-A, Fetal Alcohol Spectrum Disorder in the Criminal Justice System, August 14-15, 2010.

16 LaDue R, Dunne T. Capacity concerns and Fetal Alcohol Syndrome. *The FEN Pen* Winter 1996; 2-3.

17 LaDue R, Dunne T. Fetal Alcohol Syndrome: Implications for sentencing in the criminal justice system. *The FEN Pen* Fall 1996; 2-3.

18 LaDue R, Dunne T. Fetal Alcohol Syndrome: Implications for sentencing in the criminal justice system. *The FEN Pen* Spring 1997; 2-3.

19 *R. v. Harper,* 2009 YKTC 18, 2009. Territorial Court of Yukon, His Honou Judge Heino Lilles.

20 *U.S. v Root,* 2009. U.S. District Court, District of Colorado, Hon. John L. Kane.

21 *Hall v. Florida,* 2014, U.S. Supreme Court, No. 12 – 10882., Opinion by Justice Kennedy

22 LaDue R, Dunne T. Issues in the legal realm: Fetal Alcohol Syndrome and the decision to decline or retain. *The FEN Pen* Spring 1996; 2-6.

23 Conry JL, Fast DK. Fetal alcohol syndrome and the criminal justice system. Vancouver, BC: Fetal Alcohol Syndrome Resources Society, 2000.

24 Cox LV, Clairmont D, Cox S. Knowledge and attitudes of criminal justice professionals in relation to fetal alcohol spectrum disorder, *Canadian Journal of Clinical Pharmacology* 2008;15;e306-e313.

25 Streissguth A. Unpublished manuscript.

26 Prendergast M, Podus D, Finney J, Greenwell L, Roll J. Contingency Management for Treatment of Substance Use Disorders: A Meta-Analysis.

Addiction 2006;101:1546-1560.

27 http://www.ndrn.org/en/about/paacap-network.html

28 Marlatt GA, Parks GA, Kelly KA. Monograph Series 9 National Drug Court Institute. Quality Improvement for Drug Court: Evidence-Based Practices. National Drug Court Institute 2008;23-32.

29 SAMHSA FASD Center for Excellence Web site: http://www.fasdcenter.samhsa.gov/.

30 Illinois Compiled Statutes, ch. 775, section 5/11a-2.

CHAPTER 8

Communications

THE DANGERS OF CYBERSPACE

Ira J. Chasnoff, M.D., and Jonathan Leuchs, M.P.I.A.

Adolescents with FASDs are at special risk as they face the expanding digital world. Smartphones, "sexting," and social networks pose dangerous pitfalls for all teens, but especially for those with poor judgment, impulsivity, and difficulties connecting actions and consequences due to prenatal alcohol exposure. In this chapter dealing with technology and connectivity, specific suggestions are provided for protecting adolescents from dangerous connections in cyberspace.

Parenting is more difficult today than ever. In addition to the usual sharp curves and detours that all parents face when trying to guide their child on the journey to adulthood and adult competency, the Internet and its associated media have thrown up potential minefields that even ten years ago were unimaginable. Today's adolescents are developing in an environment in which they're bombarded with the message that sharing everything online is a social necessity (blogs, social networking sites, photo-sharing sites), and where many celebrities playfully "sext" their lives for public consumption.

BRAIN-BASED DECISION-MAKING

To appreciate how easily an adolescent can become entangled in various traps that lie waiting in the cyberworld, it is necessary to understand normal brain development and decision-making at this stage of development. As a child transitions into adolescence, physical and hormonal changes provide an overlay[1] to the young person's becoming more reflective of her self and developing a greater capacity to think and manage increasingly complex concepts. Thus the adolescent becomes more strategically minded[2] as her brain, in particular the amount of white matter, is growing rapidly. The most prominent structure made of white matter is the corpus callosum, which connects separate areas of the left and right cortex.[3] The corpus callosum integrates the two cerebral hemispheres, and therefore functions to unify sensory fields, storing and retrieving memories, and focusing attention.[3]

    The prefrontal cortex and the parietal cortex are two other regions of the brain that have been shown with MRI imaging to continually develop during adolescence. This growth affects executive functions, which in general improve during this stage. Areas of specified attention, decision-making, response inhibition skills, ability to access multiple skills at once, all tend to improve.[2] Additionally, the development of the pre-frontal cortex affects high-level cognitive capacities like self-awareness and theory of mind.[4,5] However, a specific area of the pre-frontal cortex, the dorsolateral, does not develop completely until early adulthood. This area oversees impulse control, judgment, and decision-making.

During this period of rapid brain development, the adolescent experiences concomitant development in the processing of social emotions. Social emotions are those that require representation of mental state, such as embarrassment, guilt, shame, and pride. As social emotions develop around the time of puberty, adolescents become more aware of and concerned with people's opinions of them, and the notion of self begins to depend more and more on perceived social reputation.[6] This ability to process social emotions continues to develop into adulthood. As the adolescent's brain, and therefore his mental and social emotional functions, is developing rapidly, he has limited capacity for self-regulation and high susceptibility to peer pressure.

THE INTERNET AND CONNECTEDNESS

Because adolescents are in this transitional stage of rapid cognitive and social emotional development, they are at increased risk for harmful behavior while using and exploring the Internet and social media. The Internet and social media, at their essence, connect and integrate users, and provide them greater access to information. The Internet enhances users' ability to share their knowledge and information about themselves. One may even view the adolescent in the digital age as a socially extended mind that is distributed across the brain, body, and digital media tools.[7]

Communication on the Internet via social media becomes intimate quickly and often feels liberating for an adolescent because it can be a way to overcome shyness and feelings of self-consciousness. There can be positive effects of online communication, but those effects–a sense of well-being due to a feeling of connectedness and being liked–generally only result from communication with existing friends.[8]

Adolescents, just like adults, feel cravings for digital devices and connectivity. Digital technology has been shown to cause small spikes of dopamine in the brain, and lends itself to risky, dopamine-seeking behaviors, somewhat similar to gambling, substance abuse, or shopping, and therefore affects the mentality and brain structure of the user.[9] Adolescents are especially susceptible to the addictive nature of the Internet, and the concurrent problem of sleep deprivation.[10]

As an example, Sid Gardner, author of Chapter 6, offers a perspective on an aspect of technology that is often overlooked, but can have significant deleterious effects: networked video games.

> *We use the word addiction with care. But our adopted son Rob, diagnosed in childhood with ARND, became addicted, pure and simple, to video games. He would stay up all night playing multiplayer online games, amassing points in the deliberate entrapment that game designers use to keep their customers coming back over and over. He refused dinner, his room deteriorated well below the usual bear den standards of adolescent males, and he "forgot" his household chores more often than he remembered them. To be sure, there was a balancing plus that came with all these minuses—Rob turned out to be a natural online leader, with a dozen or so players following his lead in some of the games. But the net effect was terrible for his school work, and sapped his will to study in his first set of college classes. And then, after some interventions that involved taking his computer away and telling him he could not live with us if he didn't curb his addiction, he made it through the withdrawal.*

Peer acceptance and interpersonal feedback regarding self-identity, both of which are prominent features of social network sites,[11] are important predictors of adolescent self-esteem and well-being. Rob received this positive reinforcement from his connectedness to other players and his mastery of his digital device.

THE INTERNET AND RISK OF SELF

The disinhibiting nature of the Internet and online communication can often lead to hostile, insulting, and overwhelming interactions between Internet users. Inhibition is lost when there are no non-verbal cues to guide communication and interaction.[11] Unfortunately, research is showing that adolescents' behavior online and through digital, mobile devices can translate into negative "offline" behavior, such as cyberbullying, privacy encroachment, and sexting. As recipients of these behaviors, for adolescents who receive nothing but negative feedback when they put themselves out in the cyberworld for all to see, the decrease in their self-esteem from engaging on social media can be overwhelming and harmful.[12]

Friend networking sites encourage participants to form relationships and to comment on one another's appearance and personality. Users' self-esteem can easily become wrapped up in feedback they receive from friends on the site, many of whom they have never met. In one study,[12] adolescents' self-esteem was affected solely by the tone of the feedback that they received on their profiles: positive feedback enhanced adolescents' self-esteem, and negative feedback decreased their self-esteem. For most teens, the feedback they receive on their profiles almost always is positive. For these adolescents, the use of friend networking sites may be an effective vehicle for enhancing their self-esteem. However, for a teen who is perceived by peers as "different" or "not with it," as is frequently the case for adolescents with FASDs, comments on their profiles may be devastating.

THE INTERNET, SOCIAL MEDIA, AND ADOLESCENTS WITH FASDs

If you've read closely, by this point you realize that every chapter has addressed the problems of poor judgment, lack of inhibition, not comprehending consequences of behavior, being easily led by peers, and myriad other behavioral deficits that characterize the lives of adolescents affected by prenatal alcohol exposure. These deficits are magnified when the disinhibition allowed by the Internet enters the equation.

Jenna is 14 years old, a lovely young lady with ARND. She is bright, social, and eager to please. Without hesitation, she sent nude photographs of herself to her "14 year-old boyfriend" that she met on the Internet. When her parents discovered the pictures, they immediately called the police. The police came to the house and arrested Jenna for the distribution of child pornography. Of course, it was a ploy by the police to force Jenna to give them information about her "boyfriend," but once they realized that Jenna knew nothing about him except for his email address, the charges were dropped.

Parents should understand that any digital media shared, especially photos, can, and likely will, be displayed publicly. Meanwhile, adolescents and teens have a difficult time appreciating how inappropriate types of images can be misused by their peers, much in the way kids in high school fail to appreciate the dangers of drinking and driving. Parents need to be aware that, at worst, a child can be prosecuted for obscenity, or even child pornography, if he or she was producing and distributing homemade sexual videos. Teens are also vulnerable to bullying and cyberbullying as a result of sharing compromising information (e.g., photos). Widespread redistribution of private images can lead to severe emotional trauma, physical injury, and even suicide.

Given the best of circumstances with the best of well-regulated children, the challenges and dangers posed by social media, unfettered access to a world of both positive and negative information, and instant communication that is next to impossible to delete, even the most attentive and well-meaning parents are going to have to deal with potential calamities. But for children and adolescents with FASDs, their neurobehavioral deficits and challenges make them especially vulnerable to exploitation and injudicious, inappropriate, and, perhaps, illegal activity.

Carol Hurley, the author of Chapter 5 in this book, shares her experience with managing her young adult daughter's access to the wide world of cyberspace:

> *After that incident I went online with my cell phone provider and reallocated the data for our phones. I allowed her phone only the minimum data and moved the rest of it over to my line. She then had insufficient data to text or email photographs. She did continue to take selfies and try to send them, but was never able to. The rule in my home was has always been if you live here, I am paying your bills, so I get to know all of the passwords. The moment a password changes without my knowledge, I pick up the device in question and keep it until the passwords are forthcoming. Once again, it isn't pretty- and there are many arguments, but I have to prevail. My child's safety and survival depend on it.*
>
> *I have GPS tracking installed on our cell phones, so at any moment I can see exactly where my child is. When I am not home I disable the wireless internet connection in our home so I can monitor access and inappropriate content cannot be accessed.*

Carol, Sid, and other parents of adolescents with FASDs have to be especially vigilant in monitoring and controlling their children's access to the Internet and social media. Due to the impulsive behavior found in so many of these young people affected by prenatal alcohol exposure, the opportunity to engage in an activity, regardless of consequences, is too much for them to ignore. Easily led by more sophisticated peers, the young person engages in activities that do not really "make sense:"

- Carrying on inappropriate on-line conversations even when likelihood of being detected is high
- Impulsive, opportunistic activities with no appreciation of consequences
- No exit strategy for when even they can tell something is going wrong
- Frank conversations, providing information they think is being looked for
- No apparent guilt or remorse

- Unable to appreciate magnitude or implications of inappropriate activities.

There are some simple, and some not so simple, steps parents can take to protect their child:
- Check to see if one or more file sharing software packages have been installed on your child's computer.
- Before agreeing to purchase a new electronic device, ask her to explain it, and how she plans to use it.
- Whenever possible, keep computers in common, open spaces. Set and keep rules about using phones and tablets while at home – out of bedrooms
- Keep all family phones together while charging at night
- Conduct inspections of mobile devices - privacy is a privilege, not a right
- Review an adolescent's email and text messages while he or she is sitting beside you and have ongoing discussions about appropriate conversations and online activity
- Control data usage on smart phones
- Use surveillance software on a computer to: monitor web activity, including emails, instant messaging, chat, web browsing and file downloads
- Collaborate and interact: require full "Friend" status on all social networking sites: cyber-supervising
- Require that the child shares passwords on any device and/or social network
- Physically (as opposed to online, 'social') network with friends and teachers to stay abreast of what is and may be happening.

The Internet is a grand source of information and can provide a young person with positive links to others. However, a parent of an adolescent, especially an adolescent with FASDs, must exercise continuous diligence and oversight, balancing the good of the Internet and its omnipresence in the world of the teen with the potential for harm.

NOTES

1   Rutler and Rutler, *Developing Minds,* Penguin, London, 1993.

2   Blakemore SJ, Choudhury S. Development of the Adolescent Brain: Implications for the Executive Function and Social Cognition: *Journal of Child Psychology and Psychiatry,* 2006;47:3/4, 296-312.

3   Lenroot RK, Giedd JN. Brain development in children and adolescents: Insights from anatomical magnetic resonance imaging, *Neuroscience and Biobehavioral Reviews,* 2006;30:718-729.

4   Ochsner, Current Directions in Social Cognitive Neuroscience, *Current Opinion in Neurobiology,* 2004;14:254-258.

5   Frith, Frith, Development and Neurophysiology of Mentalizing, *Philosophical Transactions of the Royal Society of London: Series B, Biological Sciences,* 2003;358(1431):459–473.

6   Burnet S, Bird G, Moll J, Frith C., Blakemore SJ, Development During Adolescence of the Neural Processing of Social Emotion, *Journal of Cognitive Neuroscience* 2009;21(9):1736-1750.

7   Clark, Chalmers The Extended Mind, *Analysis,* 2003;58(1):7-19.

8   Valkenburg PM, Jochen P. Social Consequences for the Internet for Adolescents: A Decade of Behavior, *Current Directions in Psychological Science* 2009;18:1.

9   Small, Vorgan, *iBrain: Surviving the technological alteration of the modern mind,* New York, HarperCollins, 2008.

10   Clinical Report - The Impact of Social Media on Children, Adolescents, and Families, American Academy of Pediatrics, Pediatrics, 2011, www.pediatrics.org/cgi/doi/10.1542/peds.2011-0054.

11   Harter, *The Construction of the Self: A Developmental Perspective,* New York, Guilford Press, 1999.

12   Valkenburg PM, Peter J, Schouten AP. Friend Networking Sites and their Relationship to Adolescents' Well-Being and Social Self-Esteem, *Cyberpsychology & Behavior,* 2006;9(5):584-590.

Author Biographies

Ira J. Chasnoff, MD is president of NTI Upstream and a professor of clinical pediatrics at the University of Illinois College of Medicine in Chicago. He is one of the nation's leading researchers in the field of prenatal exposure to alcohol and illicit drugs and the author of eight books, including *Drugs, Alcohol, Pregnancy, and Parenting,* which received the Book of the Year Award from the American Journal of Nursing. He lives in Chicago, IL.

Julie Kable, PhD is an Assistant Professor in the Department of Psychiatry and Behavioral Sciences and is a licensed pediatric psychologist who has over 20 years of experience working with children with neurodevelopmental disabilities with a particular focus on children with a history of prenatal alcohol exposure. She was the 2013 President of the Fetal Alcohol Spectrum Disorder Study Group, a professional organization dedicated to scientific inquiry into the etiology of fetal alcohol syndrome (FAS), the characteristics of Fetal Alcohol Spectrum Disorders (FASDs), and methods to improve the lives of individuals with FASDs. Her work has involved both research and the clinical care of children with FASDs. Dr. Kable is also the Assistant Director of the Emory Neurodevelopmental Exposure and Fetal Alcohol and Drug Exposure Clinics. She has been instrumental in the development of innovative interventions for children with FASDs that focus on improving self-regulation, early math skills and adaptive living skills. In addition to her intervention research, she has participated in several prospective longitudinal studies on the impact of various teratogens (i.e. alcohol, cigarettes, cocaine) on development throughout the lifespan, including studies using neuroimaging procedures with adults who were prenatally exposed to alcohol. Dr. Kable has also served on expert panels related to the identification and care of individuals with FASDs.

Sidney Gardner serves as President of Children and Family Futures, Inc. He served as Director of the Center for Collaboration for Children at California State University, Fullerton from 1991 – 2001. He is the author of Beyond Collaboration to Results, published by Arizona State University, which assesses the recent history of community collaboratives in the context of the growing move toward results-based accountability. His four-stage model of the developmental life cycle of collaboratives has been used extensively throughout the nation, along with a self-assessment instrument for collaboratives and a Collaborative Values Inventory designed to assess the degree of consensus on underlying values within a collaborative. Mr. Gardner's book, "Cities, Counties, Kids, and Families: the Essential Role of Local Government" (2005), describes a model for developing strategic policy for children and family policy in local governments.

Ronald J. Powell, PhD is the director of the Desert Mountain SELPA in San Bernardino, California. He has been a leading advocate for special education services for children and youth with FASD and has integrated clinical and educational strategies to best serve these young people.

Jenae Holtz is the Director of The Desert/Mountain Children's Center in Apple Valley, California. She is a Licensed Marriage, Family Therapist. Jenae has worked with children, adolescents and their families for the past 30 years in the mental health field. These experiences range from private clinical practice, school-based therapy, group homes and psychiatric hospitals. Jenae has been an administrator in the mental health field at various times through her career specializing in children and adolescences.

Jenae currently oversees the Desert/Mountain Children's Center which serves over 6,000 children and youth annually. This center provides services for over 22,000 square miles in the High Desert of Southern California. This region if often very rural, has pockets of extreme poverty and is a high intensity drug trafficking area. As such her center, in addition to providing traditional mental health services, has developed specialized skills in serving the traumatized and drug and alcohol endangered child.

Jenae is committed to providing services to children and 'doing' whatever it takes to attain the necessary interventions. Her concern for our at-risk children is evidenced by her commitment to developing or attaining specialized services.

Carole Hurley became licensed as a foster parent for the State of Texas in the mid-1990s. Six months later the light of her life toddled in the front door, and Carole's life was forever changed. Her career evolved from a general litigation private law practice, to managing federal grant programs that worked with judges and child welfare stakeholders throughout the state to improve how children moved through the child protection system and to enhance outcomes for at-risk children and families. Seven years later, a drug and alcohol exposed newborn was placed in Carole's home, and once again both her personal and professional life took a turn. Eventually both daughters received diagnoses indicative of prenatal alcohol exposure, and Carole's work with children in care and the courts began to focus on the challenges of the prenatally exposed population.

In the ensuing years Carole has represented children in foster care who have special, complex behavioral, educational, and mental health challenges, been a frequent public speaker on the topic of prenatal alcohol exposure and the courts, and has provided training on behavior management and academic issues to foster and adoption providers. In 2007, she received the State Bar of Texas Fairy Davenport Rutland Award for Distinguished Service to Children and Families.

In 2013, Carole became the Chief Administrative Law Judge for the Texas Health and Human Services Commission. She is Chair of the State Bar Committee on Child Abuse and Neglect, Chair of the Travis County Child Protective Services Board, and is a member of the Texas Fetal Alcohol Spectrum Disorders (FASD) Prevention Task Force. Her most important job, though, is being Kara and Emma Hurley's mom.

Howard Davidson. J.D. has been actively involved with the legal aspects of child protection for 40 years. He has directed the American Bar Association's *Center on Children and the Law,* leading a twenty person staff in work on child welfare law and policy improvement, since its 1978 establishment.

He' s served as chair of the U.S. Advisory Board on Child Abuse and Neglect, is a founding board member of the National Center for Missing and Exploited Children, and is also on the governing boards of ECPAT-USA, a national group focused on law and policy reform related to child trafficking and sexual exploitation, and the National Foster Care Coalition. He recently served on a National Academy of Sciences/Institute of Medicine Child Maltreatment Panel and is an advisor to the National Center for the Review & Prevention of Child Deaths.

He has led ABA efforts to address the topic of Fetal Alcohol Spectrum Disorders, developing the text and securing cosponsors for an ABA-approved FASD policy resolution and report, and a half-day ABA continuing legal education program on FASD. He also worked with the U.S. Department of Justice's Office of Juvenile Justice and Delinquency Prevention to plan and convene an invitational Listening Session on justice system improvement for children, youth and families affected by FASD. Howard's local work includes membership on Maryland Children's Justice Act Committee and being named by the Mayor of Philadelphia to a Community Oversight Board helping guide improvements in that city's child protection system. Howard also was selected as a U.S. delegate to the first World Congress Against the Commercial Sexual Exploitation of Children.

Kathyrn A. Kelly has spent more than 30 years of her career working in the juvenile and criminal justice systems, including serving as a Mitigation Specialist/Investigator representing California Death Row inmates seeking review of their capital sentences.

Realizing that many of her Death Row clients were living with brain damage that could be attributed to their prenatal alcohol exposure, in 2001, Ms. Kelly co-founded the FASD Legal Issues Resource Center for which she has served as director since its inception. Through this work, Ms. Kelly has developed a website that summarizes state and federal court cases in which FASDs is an issue and has trained criminal and juvenile justice and addiction professionals in the U.S., Canada, U.K., Northern Ireland, Iceland, Norway, Sweden, Portugal, Spain, New Zealand, Australia and the Netherlands.

Ms. Kelly works, daily and worldwide, with parents, caregivers, service providers and attorneys, on cases involving children, adolescents and adults living with FASDs who are in trouble with the law.

Discussion Questions

CHAPTER 1

**FETAL ALCOHOL SPECTRUM DISORDERS:
BEHAVIOR BELONGS IN THE BRAIN**

1. Why is it so difficult to find out if a pregnant woman is drinking alcohol? What strategies do you think would work to make gathering this kind of information a normal part of prenatal care? What kind of public prevention campaigns do you think would work to prevent alcohol use during pregnancy?
2. Whose job is it to diagnose a child with Fetal Alcohol Syndrome or any of the other clinical conditions within the fetal alcohol spectrum? What are the professional disciplines that should be involved in assessment and diagnosis? How could a team of clinicians best put together an assessment approach that would benefit the alcohol-exposed child?
3. The DSM-5 has presented a new diagnostic term for individuals affected by prenatal alcohol exposure: Neurodevelopmental Disorder with Prenatal Alcohol Exposure (ND-PAE). Do you think this will help professionals and families access care for children and youth with Fetal Alcohol Spectrum Disorders (FASDs)? How has the varying terminology over the past 40 years affected assessment, diagnosis, and access to services for individuals with prenatal alcohol exposure?
4. Does it really make a difference if a child with FASDs is not diagnosed or is diagnosed incorrectly? How does it affect the approach to intervention and treatment?
5. How does the concept of behavioral teratology fit with understanding the long-term outcome of children and youth with FASDs? Why is this an important consideration?

CHAPTER 2

FETAL ALCOHOL SPECTRUM DISORDERS IN THE TEENAGE YEARS

6. How can parents know when an adolescent's behavior is due to the effects of prenatal alcohol exposure and when the behavior is just part of normal adolescent development?
7. Can you give some examples of behaviors that a teen might demonstrate

on a day-to-day basis as a result of problems with neurocognitive functioning? What about self-regulation problems and difficulties with adaptive functioning?

8. Why do you think problems with executive functioning are mentioned so frequently throughout this book? What implications do deficits in executive functioning have across the life span for the individual affected by prenatal alcohol exposure?

9. What are some ways in which "peer pressure" can be especially negative for the teen with FASDs? Can "peer pressure" ever be put to good use? How?

CHAPTER 3

FASDs, ADOLESCENCE AND SCHOOL

1. How can the Individuals with Disabilities Education Act be used to support children and youth with FASDs? What are the barriers?
2. Why do teachers so frequently view children with prenatal alcohol exposure as if the child has attention deficit disorder (ADD)? How does it make a difference in the classroom approach to learning?
3. What aspects of "direct instruction" do you think meet the needs of children and youth with FASDs?
4. What steps can a school and a family take to create a "school/home bridge" in order to best serve the needs of the child affected by prenatal alcohol exposure?

CHAPTER 4:

THE PERFECT STORM: COMPLEXITY OF SEXUAL BEHAVIORS IN ADOLESCENTS WITH FASDs

1. What are the differences between addressing sexual development and sexuality in teens with FASDs and the approach for typically developing teens? Why do you think a different approach is needed?
2. Have you seen a teen with FASDs who got "stuck" at an earlier developmental level when it came to understanding sexuality? Describe the teen's behavior. What do you think is the best approach for addressing

this problem?

3. What are the circumstances that place teens with FASDs in special danger, both from a victim and a perpetrator perspective? What can you do to protect the child, adolescent and young adult with FASDs?

CHAPTER 5:
S.O.S: A PARENT'S CRY FOR HELP OR A SURVIVAL STRATEGY?

1. What elements of Kara's story fit with what the other chapters have addressed? How do you see the brain-based behaviors expressed through Kara's day-to-day functioning?
2. What steps has Carole taken in order to support Kara throughout her childhood and adolescence? What has worked, and what has not worked?
3. What does Carole mean by "S.O.S.?" If you have a child with FASDs, what are the elements of S.O.S. that can be incorporated into your family's lifestyle? If you are a professional working with families who are raising a child with FASDs, what recommendations can you make?
4. Will Kara's story eventually have a happy ending? Why or why not?

CHAPTER 6:
FETAL ALCOHOL SPECTRUM DISORDERS, ADOLESCENTS, AND THE CHILD WELFARE SYSTEM

1. How well does the child welfare system in your state serve children and youth with FASDs? What kind of information exists to help you answer this question?
2. How does the issue of behavioral teratology, discussed in Chapter 1, come into play when considering children and youth who have been placed in the child welfare system?
3. What are all the systems that need to work together in order to serve children and youth with FASDs who are in the child welfare system?
4. What can be done to prepare a young person for transition out of the child welfare system and into independent living?
5. What policy recommendations would you make to improve services to children and youth with FASDs who are in the child welfare system?

CHAPTER 7:
FASDs AND THE JUSTICE SYSTEM
1. What do you think are the main reasons that youth with FASDs become involved in the criminal justice system?
2. What are some strategies that parents and professionals can use to guide these very vulnerable youth away from involvement with the justice system? What approach should parents take to educating the police and local court officials about FASDs?
3. In the film, Jerry already has been arrested and jailed for three days. What do you think are the prospects for Brittany, Alison, and Kara?
4. What impact will the American Bar Association's resolution have on children and youth with FASDs? The Supreme Court recently ruled that intellectual disabilities cannot be defined by IQ but rather by cognitive functioning. How will that ruling affect children and youth with FASDs?

CHAPTER 8:
THE DANGERS OF CYBERSPACE
1. All the authors mention on-line dangers for children and youth with FASDs? Why do you think the editor felt it was necessary to include a chapter on this specific issue?
2. How do the brain-based behaviors described in previous chapters influence on-line behavior in children and youth with FASDs?
3. What are the benefits that a young person with FASDs might derive from on-line communication and social media? What are the special dangers for children and youth with FASDs when it comes to on-line communication and social media? What steps can you take to protect the young person with FASDs?